FOLLOW YOUR
TAO

Cover image by Bethan Christopher

First published in 2024 by OH
An Imprint of HEADLINE PUBLISHING GROUP

13 5 7 9 10 8 6 4 2

Cataloguing in Publication Data is available from the British Library

Hardback ISBN 978-1-80129-317-4

Printed and bound in China

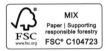

HEADLINE PUBLISHING GROUP
An Hachette UK Company
Carmelite House
50 Victoria Embankment
London EC4Y 0DZ
www.headline.co.uk
www.hachette.co.uk

OH Publisher: Lisa Dyer
Desk editor: Matt Tomlinson
Design: Lucy Palmer
Production: Arlene Lestrade

Disclaimer:
The information contained in this book is intended for educational and informational purposes only. It is not
intended to be used as a substitute for professional medical advice, diagnosis, or treatment.

Before embarking on any physical activity or incorporating the exercises provided, it is strongly recommended
to consult with a qualified healthcare professional, such as your doctor or an experienced practitioner in the
respective fields. For individuals with a history of severe trauma, it is essential to engage in the exercises under
the guidance and supervision of a qualified mental health professional or medical qigong therapist.

The author, publisher and contributors to this book shall not be held responsible for any errors, omissions or
any potential consequences arising from the use of the information provided. The reader assumes full responsibility for their actions and decisions made based on the information within this book. The use of this book
implies your acceptance of this disclaimer.

FOLLOW YOUR
TAO

A SIMPLE GUIDE TO BALACING YOUR ENERGY FOR INNER HARMONY

Stephanie Nosco

For my Dad,
who planted the seed,
and Christine,
who watered the soil

Dear Reader,

As I sit in the forest compiling the final chapters of this book, three ravens circle over my head, reminding me that publishing a book on Chinese Medicine is tricky.

It is tricky because I do not speak Chinese, nor am I of Asian descent. It is impossible to capture it fully without fluency and immersion in the Chinese culture or language. As a person of privilege, I feel humbled and honoured to have explored Eastern wisdom from a young age. However, I recognize the limitations of my perspective. Please understand that I do not claim to be a master in these topics; instead, I share this wisdom with deep curiosity, enquiry and reverence.

While this book draws its foundation from my training in qigong, Five Element theory, psychotherapy and Buddhism, it is not a repetition of what I learned, but rather an interpretation. What fills these pages is a distillation of a vast array of teachings, presented in a way that makes sense to me, and has made sense to my students and those I have sat with in therapy. This book is not meant as a religious or authoritative text on Taoism, or a textbook on Chinese medicine (as this is beyond my scope of knowledge), but rather it represents how my practice and study shine through me as I walk my Tao. I hope this perspective allows the teachings of the organs and their wisdom to be more widely accessible in a time where they are desperately needed.

There are some more traditional concepts I have left out of this book, and one or two associations that you might find categorized differently in other books on Chinese medicine. These changes were done intentionally based on my personal research, practice and experience. Due to the scope and purpose of this book, I was unable to cover the historical background of Chinese medicine in the entirety it deserves. My hope is that this book will be a starting point to your journey, and if you are called to dive deeper, you will take advantage of the resources listed in the bibliography.

May this book be of benefit to you and all human and non-human beings.
— SN

CONTENTS

INTRODUCTION
The Tao Is Like Water

'The supreme good is like water,
which nourishes all things without trying to.'

Tao Te Ching, Stephen Mitchell translation

The glacier reflects the summer sun off its icy crust, grey patches scarring its receding perimeter. I squint up and see that it is smaller and darker than I remember from childhood. Water cascades from the glacier off the rocky ledge, streaming down in multiple branches towards the lake basins below. To my left, a crowd of tourists disembark a large idling bus, their eyes focused not on the mountain, but on their phones, snapping pictures to take home with them. Despite the chaos in the parking lot, the mountain scene remains unchanged – the sound of the steady rushing water echoes like a sacred hymn through the valley.

As I sit in my car, my mind drifts to a memory of when I was 13. My father took me on an overnight hike up this mountain to the glacier. We stayed at an alpine hut, perched on the very edge of the glacial wall. I am transported to that day, when I stood on top of its snowy ledges in the middle of summer. My dad explained to me that the ice from Bow Glacier created Bow Lake, which flows as Bow River into our city before finding its way through the prairies to Hudson Bay and into the ocean.

Now, in my mid-thirties, I sit in Bow Lake parking lot wondering how long this glacier will be here, and if future generations will have the privilege of enjoying its clean waters. I roll down the window, drawing in a deep breath of mountain air mixed with the exhaust fumes from the idling bus. As I exhale, a mixture of grief and gratitude washes over me. Grief for the devastation of our planet, and gratitude for the generosity of nature despite the abuse she endures.

Not only would I not be alive without the gift of the Bow River, but in some way I can feel the spirit and wisdom of it in me. It has taught me over the years – as I have watched it, listened to it, bathed in it, drank it – something beyond what I could have learned from a book, transmitting a way of being that is in rhythm with the moon, the passing seasons and the beat of my heart.

I look over at the crowd of tourists, who are gathered in groups, posing in front of the emerald water. In their exuberance to take their photos, I sense their appreciation for the mountain and a longing for something in it they have lost. I feel myself reaching for that same thing. I appreciate the human longing to return to nature and plant it as a seed of hope in my mind. A hope that the love we have for the natural world will transpire into a new way of relating to it. I hold steady to the sound of the water that flows down the mountain, the ancient wisdom that now commands all of my attention. I shut my eyes and listen. 'The answers we need', I think, 'are in that hymn.'

You might be wondering how this anecdote has anything to do with your organs, or how following your Tao relates to the flow of water from a glacier to the sea. Let's take a moment to pause and visualize the scene I am describing in your mind's eye: water flowing down a mountain. What energy do you feel in your body as you attune to that? Can you relax into that image, just as water relaxes down a mountainside?

What you might have felt is your body unclenching and your mind moving into a state that feels familiar. You might even feel a sense of relief or more energy flowing in your body. To know the Tao, you must return, even momentarily, back to the simplicity and familiarity of nature – renounce the complexities of detail, money, relationships, time – and listen to the natural pulse of the world. Nature reminds us of the Tao because the Tao is not complicated, busy or stressed. It is the steady hum behind all creation that can be found in the sound of the river, the smell of the flower or a warm afternoon breeze.

Following your Tao is as natural as water flowing down a mountain: in its non-resistance it is generous, beautiful and deeply appreciated. Yet, praise and appreciation doesn't alter its flow. It is powerfully centred in its being without apologizing, and in doing so, nourishes the land and its creatures.

According to the theory of Chinese medicine, health – in body and in mind – depends on being in flow with our naturalness. When we resist the flow of nature, our energies become disrupted and illness arises. But when we can flow with the current of our own energy, we experience ease, which brings tremendous power – the power to create, change and heal. Following your Tao does not mean you won't suffer or go through hard times, it simply means you are flowing in the right direction, with your energies more aligned with the way nature intended.

While this book contains detailed information about your organs, their energies and emotions, the essence of it is calling you back to nature. By nature, I mean both the natural world 'out there' and your authentic spirit 'in here'. I hope through reading this book, you learn how the functioning of your organs is not separate from the elements in nature, and by attuning to the spirit of nature directly, rather than merely observing it through a photo or a car window, you inadvertently learn about the energy in your body. I also hope that by listening to your organs directly through the practices in this book, you will hear within them the spirit of nature and their wisdom as a guiding force for your life.

In a world where humanity soars above the natural world in planes, helicopters, spaceships and virtual spaces, while environmental devastation only worsens, it becomes increasingly crucial that we make a conscious effort to return to nature and rediscover the wisdom we have lost. The outer ecosystems that are in desperate need of our care are intricately connected with the systems that reside within our own bodies. As you read, I invite you to consider that your healing journey is not solely about yourself, but is a defiant act of hope and a catalyst for change within our larger ecosystem. And because you are energetically interconnected to everything in existence, by following your Tao you contribute to the healing of our planet as a whole.

WHAT IS THE TAO?

While this metaphor of the water points to the energetic essence of the Tao, in the absolute sense it cannot be named or described. It is the invisible truth that lies within and beyond all phenomena. The Tao is what creates and sustains all the laws of the universe, such as gravity and seasons, birth, death, the blossoming of flowers and the ripening of fruit. The Tao is what is holding your coffee cup together, sustaining the inner working of your organs, and illuminating the awareness behind your eyes as you read my words. It is the conscious and unconscious backdrop to your life story. It is as big as the sun and as small as an atom. The Tao can be literally translated as 'the way' and in the ultimate sense is simply: the way things are.

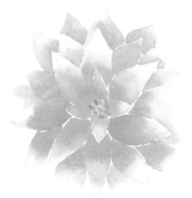

All spiritual practices are guiding us towards discovering the Tao – that is, to realize the nature of existence and the nature of our innermost selves. This discovery can bring ease to our complicated and, at times, painful lives.

The *Tao Te Ching* states that the Tao is impossible to describe and can only be experienced. And so, everything I say to you about the Tao in this book is only to awaken something deep inside you that already know. After all, Tao is the very essence of who you are at your core – interconnected to the wider web of mystery.

WHAT IS *YOUR* TAO?

Although Tao is a word to describe esoteric truths of ultimate reality, it can also be used to describe the essential energetic pattern of something. For example, it is the nature of water to flow with the current of gravity towards the lowest point – but it is not the nature of a tree whose branches reach against gravity towards the light. Even among trees, their nature expresses so uniquely based on the ecosystem and conditions they evolved in. Following the Tao in a relative sense means aligning ourselves with these energy currents as they express themselves within our body and mind. Nature serves as a reminder of this phenomenon. Consider the example of an oak tree; it can never transform itself into a fir tree, despite any training or education it undergoes. An oak tree remains steadfastly an oak, flowing with the current of what is, and rather than going against it out of personal will, it contributes to the larger ecosystem by simply being itself.

It can be easy to confuse your Tao with a professional career, because making money has been the focus of our collective story since the industrial revolution. 'What do you want to be when you grow up?' is a common question that kids are asked in school, which solidifies a future-oriented, economic-oriented sense of self. The Tao, however, describes a way of being that is authentic to your natural energy expression. Renowned psychiatrist Carl Jung called the process 'individuation', and used the word 'Tao' synonymously with the word 'meaning'. To follow your Tao is to live in accordance with your own meaning – to discover what kind of tree you are supposed to be and nurture its growth.

Mythologist Michael Meade names your personal Tao your 'genius'. This is inherent within you and doesn't need to be created; instead, it needs to be awakened, recognized and embraced by being true to yourself. However, as you tune yourself in to your energy, you will be able to recognize it through feeling the ease and energy it brings you. You know you are on the right track when you feel a sense of flow, as if you are going with the energy of your body as opposed to against it.

In this book, when I talk about the Tao in the ultimate sense, I am referring to the divine, the universe, God, or the essence of everything in existence. When I refer to Tao on a personal level, I am referring to your genius, and a way being that brings the most meaning, richness and expression to your life, while at the same time, giving back to the world.

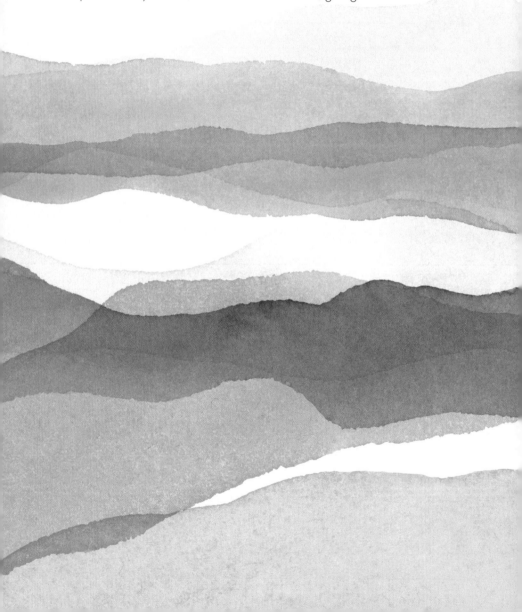

WHY LEARN ABOUT
YOUR ORGANS?

Before I began learning about Chinese medicine, my organs felt as remote to me as nature does to someone absorbed in the screen of a cellphone. Like many girls who grew up in the nineties, I learned how to relate to my body through TV and fashion magazines. These media sources often promoted the sexualization of women and emphasized the importance of having super-thin or fit bodies. I internalized the message that my body was simply an object. Despite being an athlete and maintaining a healthy diet, I approached my physical wellbeing solely as a means to optimize my body's performance, treating it like a well-oiled machine. Even my yoga practice, at first, became just another project to improve my body.

   In my early adulthood, I was lost. I sought validation and guidance externally, leading me to drift into jobs that seemed devoid of meaning and relationships that left me unsatisfied. I grappled with an inherent feeling of being an imposter, leading a life that didn't truly belong to me. I also was sick a lot, despite being young and otherwise 'healthy'. Only upon reflection do I realize that the distance I sensed from my life was mirrored by the disconnection I had with my body.

   When I started learning the language of the organs and their spirits, the relationship I had with myself changed. My organs were no longer inanimate lumps of flesh inside my torso, but alive vessels of wisdom I could turn to for guidance. I started treating my body like a living, breathing, animate creation, deserving of respect. In a mysterious listening exchange, my body began to guide me, without using reason or rationality, towards a life rich with meaning and deep purpose. As my energetic vibration shifted, my outer circumstances also began to change. While I am still human and struggle as everyone does, I am more in tune with the intelligent forces guiding me from the inside, and as a result have stepped into a life that is better suited for my energy. I am able to listen to my own authority and surround myself with people and conditions that support my flourishing. I waiver less with voices outside that tell me what I 'should be', and walk with confidence, curiosity and wonder into what I am in the present moment.

I share this story because I know body objectification is fairly 'normal' in our culture. My hope is that as you read this book, you can also attune to this deeper listening and that it helps you step in sync with the life you, and only you, were meant to live.

This book will also offer another way to look at stress. Stress is a leading cause of numerous diseases, and even premature death. Unfortunately, doctors lack the time to discuss the intricate details of the stress or emotions that are at the root of the issue. What I admire about the Chinese energetic model is that the mind-body connection is not a vague concept, but has been meticulously observed and documented over thousands of years. The earliest surviving work on Chinese medicine, *Huangdi Neijing Su Wen*, left behind a detailed map of how stress is held and stored within the body, and how different organs are influenced by certain emotions. Equipped with this map, 'listening to the body' takes on a whole new meaning. It becomes an active and participatory process, rather than an abstract notion. This book offers a simplification of that map as a way to better take care of your health, because it is one thing to go to acupuncture or massage, but another thing to be an active agent for the prevention of stress, and therefore the prevention of disease.

THE TAO IS LIKE WATER

QI: THE DANCE
OF YIN AND YANG

From the Taoist cosmological perspective, the universe as you know it appeared out of the unknowable, ultimate Tao. There were no elements, seasons, plants, animals, people or movement. Mysteriously, this amorphous space divided into the polarities of heaven and earth, or what is referred to in Chinese medicine as yin and yang.

Yin is the passive principle related with matter, the feminine, dark, damp, heavy, and the moon and earth; while yang is the active principle related to the ephemeral, masculine, bright, light, dry, and the sun. Just as the negative and positive charges create a magnetic field, the division of yin and yang created the energetic field known as 'qi'.

Qi (pronounced 'chee'), often translated as 'energy', is the invisible, animating force of the universe that nourishes life and sustains its movement. Qi is everywhere – in our bodies, in the food we eat and in the air we breathe. Qi exists at different densities depending on how much yin and how much yang it is expressing within it.

As a universal law, masculine principal moves towards feminine, negative ions move towards positive ones, and higher pressure moves towards lower pressure; that is, yin is always moving towards yang, and yang is always moving towards yin – it is the tension between the two that creates movement. You can observe the movement of yin and yang in a season: spring is the movement of yin to yang with summer being the apex of yang (the light); autumn is the movement of yang back to yin, with the winter solstice being the pinnacle of yin (the dark). You can observe these yin/yang cycles within an arc of a breath, a day and a lifetime – everything in the universe is moving through cycles of expansion (yang) and contraction (yin).

When it comes to the body, your qi flows through energy channels known as meridians. Yin energy flows up the inside lines of your body from your feet to your head, while the yang energy flows down the outside of your body from your head to your feet. Even though yin is represented by the earth and yang by the heavens, both energies flow towards their opposite: yin is in the process of becoming yang, while yang is in the process of becoming yin.

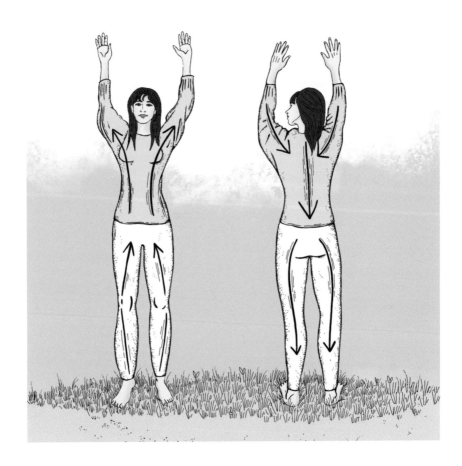

The concepts of yin and yang are important to understand for three reasons. Firstly, they lay the foundations for you to understand the categorization of organs described in detail in this book. Your body has five yin (zang) organs (kidneys, heart, lungs, liver and spleen) and five yang (fu) organs, (bladder, small intestine, large intestine, gallbladder and stomach), with each yin organ being paired with a yang organ. Yin organs are solid, and are primarily responsible for producing and storing qi, blood and body fluids. The yang organs are hollow and are primarily responsible for digesting and moving nutrients through the body. The theory of yin and yang helps explain why two seemingly unrelated organs, such as the small intestine and the heart, work together: each organ needs an opposing yang force to balance the flow of its qi.

Secondly, yin and yang help describe how qi exists at different densities – consciousness, spirit and the mind are the most yang aspects of qi, while matter and physicality are the most yin (densest) aspects of qi. The organ energies also contain a different amount yin or yang qi, with the kidneys being the most yin in nature, associated with winter, and the heart being the most yang in nature, associated with summer. Knowing the nature of yang and yin, will help you get to know the quality of the qi that is flowing in your body and mind.

Lastly, yin and yang represent two very different aspects of qi that you can seek to harmonize in your daily life. In general, yang is expressed by activities that are fast moving and external, such as expression, extroversion and mental activity; while yin is expressed and nourished by slower moving, introverted actives that promote deep embodied experiences. Even without knowing any details about the organ energies, becoming more balanced in your yin and yang activities can help to harmonize your qi.

For example, meditation would be a relatively yin activity, as the body is more passive, while going for a run would be a yang activity, with the body being more active. Attending a staff party on a Friday night would be more yang because it requires more energy to be external, while staying in and watching a movie would be more yin (internal). Neither of these activities is inherently better than the other, but can be helpful or harmful depending on your energy at that time. If you have been sitting all day at work, doing a seated meditation might not be the activity that will bring you back to balance; instead, going for a run would bring more yang activity to the mind and body to bring you back to balance. The principles of yin and yang teach us that there is no one prescription for balance – rather, it is about tuning these currents of yin and yang through the seasons of the year and the seasons of your life, all the while seeking to step in harmony with your Tao.

WHAT IS CHINESE MEDICINE?

Chinese medicine has evolved over thousands of years. The Wu Yi, primarily women in the communities, were shamanic healers who treated various ailments, including medical, psychological and spiritual disharmonies. Influenced by centuries of patriarchal rule and strict political regimes, Chinese medicine has lost much of these spiritual and mythical roots, but despite this, its holistic foundations have remained. Unlike Western medicine, which sees the body as a machine with parts that need 'fixing', Chinese medicine perceives the body as a dynamic and interconnected ecosystem. It focuses on rebalancing the vital energies within this ecosystem rather than treating isolated symptoms. This whole-body approach addresses the underlying energetic imbalances that contribute to the development of diseases.

While acupuncture needles may come to mind when thinking of Chinese medicine, it's important to note that acupuncture is just one branch of Chinese medicine. The other branches include herbalism, massage and qigong. All these holistic therapies have the same aim: to bring the body's ecosystem back into balance.

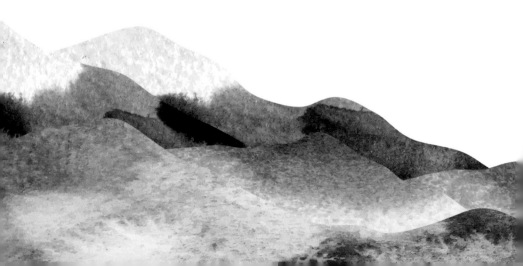

WHAT IS QIGONG?

As you have learned, the word 'qi' means energy, while 'gong' refers to skilful work. Therefore, 'qigong' involves skilful work done to move, balance and harmonize energy.

There are three main categories of qigong: marital qigong, which is done with the intention of physical strength and self-defense; medical qigong, which is practiced with the intention of maintaining health; and spiritual qigong, which is done with the intention to awaken. Within these three schools, there are thousands of different exercises, philosophies, techniques and opinions of what, how and why to practice.

This book is inspired by the medical qigong branch and its emphasis on the mind–body connection through the mind and emotions. It is helpful to understand that medical qigong is not limited to exercises but refers to an entire healing modality. This includes meditations, therapeutic ways to move emotions, healing sound therapies and treatments similar to reiki or cranial sacral therapy.

Qigong, among the various branches of Chinese medicine, is one of the oldest and most widely practiced methods in China for maintaining health. Before the 1950s, health maintenance practices were referred to as 'Dao Jia Yang Sheng Shu' ('Daoist Arts of Nurturing Life'). Qijong gained popularity in the 1950s as a means of preserving ancient healing arts and distinguishing them as a form of medicine rather than a religious practice; this helped safeguard these practices from potential destruction during the political regime at that time. Ken Cohen's seminal book *The Way of Qigong* (Random House, 1997) also made qijong and Taoism more popular.

This understanding emphasizes that while termed 'medical qigong', the practices primarily revolve around life preservation and restoring balance, rather than focusing solely on curing diseases, as is typical in Western medicine. Originally, the concept of 'nurturing life' encompassed spiritual practices and engaged with all aspects of the mind, illustrating a holistic approach to wellbeing.

How to move your qi

Below are the four main ways energy is moved, and we will be using these in the exercises that you'll find throughout this book.

1. **Movement** This includes qigong forms, but energy will also be moved by stretching, yoga, walking and any mechanical force that is applied to the body, such as acupuncture needles or massage.
2. **Breath** There are many different breathing techniques used in qigong, and some very basic ones will be described in this book. Breath directly impacts our qi through activating or deactivating our autonomic nervous system. It also helps to circulate the qi throughout the body.
3. **Intention** There is a popular saying within the qigong teachings that 'qi follows yi'. Yi (pronounced 'yee') is our intention – qi will always flow where the intention goes. In qigong practice we strengthen our intention using our imagination, to emit qi in places that are deficient, using colours to emit certain frequencies. This concept will be further explored in the chapters of this book.
4. **Sound** Sound is vibration and is a very powerful way to move qi. There are certain sounds that resonate with each organ that can be healing, but be aware that sound also includes the words you say to yourself internally – and how you say them. Sound can also include music and the sounds that you surround yourself with in your daily life.

Although formal qigong practices are powerful, it is important to remember that they are only part of the equation. Because everything in this universe moves through the medium of qi, everything you do, including how you are in relationship, what foods you eat, how you spend your time and who you spend it with, where your thoughts focus, and what emotional states you embody, as well as your connection with your Tao, will all influence the movement and quality of your qi. I like to expand the definition of qigong to encompass a way of life that harmonizes qi, rather than a practice done once a week online or at a community hall.

YOU ARE THREE-DIMENSIONAL

In our current medical system, mental and physical health are typically dealt with separately. You don't visit your therapist for bladder infections or see your family doctor for counselling after a break-up. However, the division between 'mental health' and 'physical health' is relatively recent. In traditional cultures healing was seen as a holistic process; shamans and community healers addressed both the body and mind simultaneously. Healing encompassed the entire person, including their body, emotions and spirit.

Likewise, the medical qigong model recognizes you as a three-dimensional being, comprising physical, energetic and spiritual bodies. Your organs exist on these different levels, each playing a distinct role in both your physical functioning and your psyche. From the medical qigong perspective, the 'mind' that Western medicine separates from the 'body' resides within the organs themselves. Each organ is connected to specific emotions and psychological processes. Interestingly, in medical qigong the brain is not an organ in itself, and is not attributed as much to mental processing as it is in Western medicine.

When talking about organs in this book, I am not simply talking about the physical hunks of flesh that pump blood or move bile (though our organs do those things too). I am talking about interconnected energetic systems that are infused with consciousness of the Tao, the wisdom of your spirit, and of the wisdom of the earth and its billions of years of evolution. This book will not explain how organs work from an empirical perspective but uses the organs to describe the energetic conversation that is happening in your body. Our body and all of its organ systems are intelligent patterns of energy that take the shape of organs on the physical level, emotions on the energetic level, and conscious insight and inspiration on the spirit level.

Note: If you are missing one of the organs listed in this book, such as the spleen or the gallbladder, it does not mean that you do not have the energy of that organ. It might not be there on a physical level, but its energy and spirit are still present within you.

The spirit body (shen)

The spirit body is the most yang, subtle, abstract and refined aspect of qi. It doesn't have form and cannot be felt, but it illuminates, inspires and directs. The spirit body is not bound by time or space, and from a vibratory perspective has the highest frequency. When I use the term 'spirit', you may initially associate it with God, church or something otherworldly that is divorced from the practicalities of everyday life. In the context of this book, however, spirit simply refers to the conscious element of qi. Your spirit body is what shines out through your eyes and can be sensed in the field around you. It is what holds your Tao, comes to know your Tao and is expanded when you are living your Tao.

The energy body

The energy body is denser than spirit, but less dense than form. Like the spirit body, the energy body is invisible, but unlike the spirit body, it can be felt – in fact, it is defined by feeling. Every sensation you experience is your energy body talking to you. The energy body is what receives the impulses from the sense doors of the eyes, ears, nose, mouth and skin, and is what creates our desires, likes and dislikes. The energy body is what we experience life through, and is what categorizes our experiences into beauty, pain, love or tragedy. The energy body is also what drives all emotions, and is the wave that all thought surfs on. It fills your muscles with either tension or relaxation, and determines whether we clench or flow with the events of our day. It can also be related closely to aspects of our nervous system, and is greatly influenced through the power of our breath.

The energy body is the interface between the physical word and the spirit word, as well as the inner world and the outer world. You can feel this in the constant exchange of in and out in the cycle of your breath, and experience the energy body through all your emotions and sentiments about life. The energy body is always moving and exchanging information in order to establish relationships – with people, animals and your world.

The physical body

Your physical body is what you can see; you can touch it, and it has weight and density. It is the most yin out of the three bodies because it is the densest, and from a vibratory perspective it is the slowest moving. Your physical body's initial form and structure are greatly influenced by genetics and inherent physical traits, which can be difficult, if not impossible, to alter through energy work. For instance, if you are naturally short, it is unlikely that qigong or other Chinese energetic practices will help you grow taller. However, certain physical ailments that develop over time can be influenced through energy work and lifestyle modifications – we can make changes in our physical body directly through manual therapy practices such as exercise, sleep, and diet.

Thoughts and feelings influence energy and will show up as physical symptoms. Likewise, the body's health influences feelings, emotions, thoughts and actions.

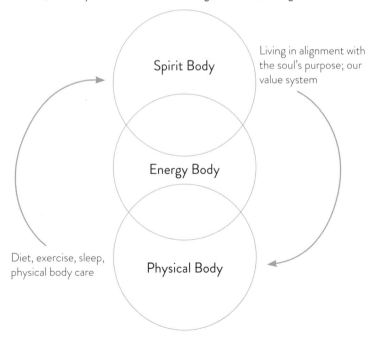

Spirit Body

Living in alignment with the soul's purpose; our value system

Energy Body

Diet, exercise, sleep, physical body care

Physical Body

Three-dimensional healing

The main thing to take away from learning about the three bodies is that they are always influencing each other. For example, working a soul-sucking job will contract your spirit body. The spirit recognizes it is out of alignment with its Tao and has no outlet to express itself. This creates feelings of frustration and agitation (qi level), which then cause you to grind your teeth at night, perhaps manifesting as locked jaw and headaches (physical level). What started at the level of spirit, now exists at the level of the physical body through the medium of emotion (qi).

While qigong may not be the best initial intervention for a broken leg or for inherited diseases or traits, it can be a tool for addressing chronic diseases that can be linked to stress levels, unprocessed trauma, or living out of alignment with your purpose. Using methods at each level –physical, emotional and spirit – will offer the most opportunity to shift the qi and to make a change. This book mainly focuses on the emotional (energy level) and psychological (spirit level) areas of healing, but please make sure you are balancing these threads I offer with physical practices and advice from nutrition experts, physiotherapists and other health care professionals to address the physical body's need as well.

THE ELEMENTS, ORGANS AND SPIRITS

Each of the five organ energies that I describe in this book – the heart, liver, spleen, lungs and kidneys – are connected energetically with an element, season, colour, direction and spirit animal, as well as with a certain sense and voice tone. These associations have been developed over centuries through careful observation of the frequencies of energy in the natural world that coincide with the frequencies within your body's inner processes. What I hope you learn from this book is that each of the elemental energies have a spiritual essence to them, which you can use as a clue to your body, its symptoms and also its wisdom.

Understanding energy in Chinese medicine is largely about recognizing patterns. Associating these elements with specific qualities helps us to create a relationship with our bodies and the natural world that is curious, playful and subjective. Getting to know some of the key correspondences will help you detect what energies might be at play in your physical, mental, emotional or spiritual body, and from there you can work to find more balance.

WHAT ARE THE FIVE SPIRITS?

Each element is animated by a spiritual essence known as the Wu Shen, which manifests within the five yin organs. The corresponding yang organs are also influenced by these spirits, and, working together, they shape our psychology. While Western medicine attributes the brain as the origin of identity, Chinese medicine perceives the psyche as being spread throughout the body, mirroring the larger cosmos.

To help understand this a bit better, I like to divide these spirit energies into upper, lower and middle spirits.

The upper spirits

The Shen and the Hun spirits, related to the heart and the liver respectively, originate from heaven. They are the most yang, and epitomize our conscious mind and altruistic capacities. Shen enters the physical body upon reception in utero, and the Hun accompanies it. Throughout our lives, the Shen and the Hun learn and develop through experiencing earthly existence. Upon death, these spirits return to heaven. Although belief in reincarnation is not necessary to benefit from the teachings in this book, the Shen and the Hun are the part of our spirit that are thought to be reborn from life to life. I often refer to them as the 'upper spirits' due to their origins from the realms above.

The middle spirit

In Taoism, the Yi is the spirit of the earth element and the stomach and spleen, and is the guardian of the space between heaven and earth. This spirit doesn't belong to heaven or earth, but rather to 'the world of man'. Here, 'man' does not refer to gender, but to all of humanity who live between the divine and earthly realms. The Yi is the spirit of intention and human volition which occurs when spirit and matter conjoin. It is both yin and yang. The Yi serves as the bridge between the upper and lower spirits, allowing one to perceive both heaven and hell, good and evil, yin and yang, and make decisions based on that understanding. When you die, the Yi is no longer active, but remains as the legacy of every accumulated action – the footprints you leave behind on this earth.

The lower spirits

The Po and the Zhi, residing in the lungs and the kidneys respectively, belong to the underworld. The development of Zhi begins in utero as the physical body forms, and the Po enters our body with our first breath. These spirits predominantly ensure survival and relate to our autonomic responses when we are afraid or aroused. They signal us to eat when we are hungry, to fight or flee when we are in danger, and also give us our sexual drives and instructs. All animals possess these spirits, carrying the wisdom of the earth within them. When you die, the Po and the Zhi will be assimilated back into the underworld.

'The Five Spirits are the Taoist map of the human psyche. The system provides a view of the nervous system and forms the basis of Chinese medical psychology.'

Lorie Eve Dechar,
The Five Spirits, 2006

WORKING WITH THE SPIRITS

In a society that leans toward dualism, there can be a tendency to pit the upper spirits against the lower spirits, classifying the upper as 'good' and the lower as 'bad'. This simplistic 'good versus evil' dichotomy leads to a fragmentation of the soul, and a disregard of the yin intuitive body knowing. This tends to happen with those on the spiritual path who are eager to develop their upper spirits (Shen and Hun) without addressing the shadows lurking in the lower spirits (Po and Zhi). Eventually, repressing these energies can cause harm internally as disease, or erupt through violence or abuse. Sadly, there are many examples of this happening among 'spiritually realized' leaders who have highly developed upper spirits but have not tended to the shadow side of impulse.

In this book, you will embark on a journey from the upper spirits, namely the heart and liver, to the organs housing the lower spirits – the lungs and kidneys. It might seem unconventional to present the organs in this order, especially for those familiar with Chinese medicine and the Five Elements cycle. By beginning our exploration with the organs infused with the most 'yang' energy and progressing towards those with the most 'yin', my intention is to facilitate a deeper integration of your spirit (light) into your bodily form (darkness). The ultimate goal is to anchor your consciousness more deeply in the physical, earthly realm, effectively grounding your mind deeper into your body.

In combination with very practical exercises and life changes listed in the soul work section in each chapter, this book will also incorporate mythical elements to help awaken certain energies that can only be stirred by this less rational, more symbolic knowing. In Chinese mythology, each organ is an archetype to your story, associated with a mythical animal. These symbolic creatures, with their vibrant colours and rich symbolism, are not to be understood as literal truths, but rather as representations of the energetic truths within you. By engaging with them, my hope is you will develop a deeper connection to your organs beyond mere intellectual understanding. This journey of self-discovery invites your imagination to play a significant role, offering you a different way of knowing and understanding yourself. Embrace this unique approach and be open to the transformative power it holds.

By exploring the five spirit energies, my intention is for you to integrate spirit into all aspects of your life, even the practical and mundane. As you descend into these depths, you will be guided to ascend with greater wisdom, self-understanding and clarity regarding your purpose and the legacy you hope to leave behind.

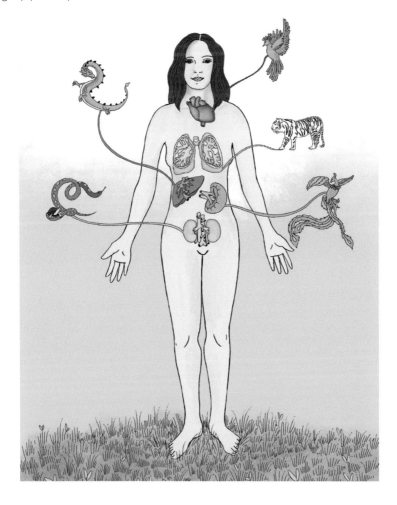

GO WITH THE FLOW

This book is structured into five chapters that correspond to the five organ energies. Each chapter consists of a theory section, providing insights into the organ's physical, energetic and spiritual functions, along with a description of common imbalances and symptoms. The chapter concludes with a soul work section, which introduces physical, energetic and spiritual practices aimed at restoring balance to that particular organ. Some of the soul work exercises only take a few minutes, while others are more extensive. Please pick exercises that work for you, and if the medicine is simply reading this book to be inspired and have more awareness about your organs, that is okay too.

My suggestion is to read the book in its entirety first and then revisit the exercises in the chapters that resonate most with the energetic imbalances you may be experiencing. You do not have to participate in each exercise on your first read-through. My hope is that the diagrams and bulleted lists can be used for quick reference and encourage you to dive deeper into certain sections. This book is also intended to support you throughout the seasons of your life, whether it be the annual seasons or the personal seasons you find yourself in. For instance, during autumn, lung energy tends to be thrown off, so you may want to return to the lung chapter during that time. Alternatively, if you are currently navigating a season of loss and transition, you might focus on the lung chapter, particularly exploring the emotional theme of letting go and grieving.

As you embark on reading this book, be attentive to the subtle vibrations within your body, as certain chapters may resonate with you or strike a chord deep within. Take your time and, most importantly, have compassion for yourself as you take this journey, never forcing or pushing yourself. Remember, water does not push its way down a mountain, it flows.

PREPARING FOR THE JOURNEY

In my work with people, I have found that the most effective approach to bringing about transformation is by genuinely acknowledging and respecting old energy patterns. It is only through self-compassion, patience and taking the time to feel into what your body is trying to say on all levels that a shift at the root is possible. The good news is that in that uprooting, it is also possible to uncover hidden desires, abilities and inclinations towards your life purpose that you didn't see before. By addressing the underlying root causes, rather than merely addressing surface symptoms, we can change our belief systems and redirect that emotional and spiritual energy towards the discovery of our potential.

My hope is that as you learn about the energetic and spiritual level of each of the organs, you begin to listen below the surface of the physical symptoms, and perhaps suspect that your recurring bladder infections are related to the insecurity you feel about your finances. You might see how suppressing your anger contributes to your pre-menstrual symptoms, or recognize that your high blood pressure is pointing to something deeper than a diet change.

As you read this book, I invite you to let go of the desire to fix your physical body. Instead, try to view its symptoms as messages from the energetic pattern in you that is asking to be transformed. Be open to the idea that your body holds all the information necessary for the next stage of your soul's development. Consider the possibility that your symptoms are the body's way of speaking to you, and that by listening you are being guided towards a way of being that your soul is longing to grow into. There is much the body knows that the conscious mind does not know. When we are in conversation with the body, including the yucky, sticky and emotional parts, we enter into a deep conversation with the hidden unconscious, and the potential energy that can propel our life into something beyond our imagining.

CHAPTER 1
Knowing Your Truth

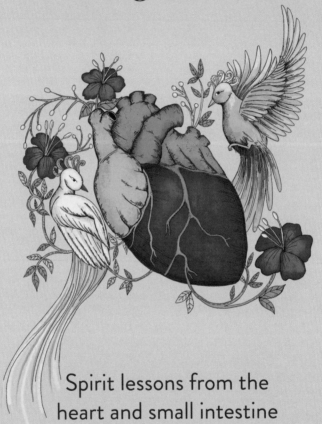

Spirit lessons from the
heart and small intestine

'The heart is the only book worth reading.'

Ajahn Chah

stretch my hands towards the fire pit, the flames lap up against the steel containment ring, like feathers of a wild bird reaching to take flight. Their warmth radiates back into my palms, sending heat up the sleeves of my cotton sweater. As my arms tire, I inch my chair closer into the circle of new friends I find myself in and the symphony of chit-chat that backgrounds the authoritative snaps of the fire. As I settle my chair into its new position, my knee almost touches the woman next to me. She looks over and smiles, her face illuminated by the moody light, painted in shadows, and her pupils reflecting the orange hues of the flame. We start to talk to acquaint ourselves and I am half present to her, and half-captivated by the mesmerizing dance of the fire, as if its flicker holds the secrets to unravel my past and guide my future.

As my eyes dart from person to person, the fire highlights something pure and genuine on their faces. I let my awareness drop from the surface content of their words to the spirit from which their words emanate. Under everything they are saying, I can appreciate the essence of each person, the fire illuminating the complexities of their individual journeys, while also highlighting the universality of our shared human longing: to be safe, to be seen and heard, to be loved. Each face is unique, yet somehow the same. I linger in this reflection, feeling gratitude for the human spirit. Then, I open myself more fully to the conversation and the joy of the circle, my heart warming to the group, and my belly filling with laughter.

Related to the element of fire, the season of summer and the voice tone of laughter, the heart is where relationships are born. It gives us the invaluable feelings of joy, peace and a deep sense of belonging to ourselves, others and nature. As the receptacle of light, the heart is home to the most enduring aspect of ourselves, namely our Shen, which can be likened to pure consciousness.

While spirit lives in the vessels of all organs, the illumination of the Shen is the thread that runs through all of the spirit energies, connecting them to the Divine.

The spirit animal of the heart is the vermilion bird, whose delicate wings require space to rest and breathe. The heart becomes overwhelmed by shock and too much noise, and so it requires time for prayers, introspection and solitude. The Shen easily lifts out of the body without this quiet time – like fire, it requires as much space as it does fuel.

The heart also contains within it your individuality and the personal truths that you must defend through setting boundaries with others, and it encourages greater connection through more authenticity in relationships. Related to the south direction and the sun's blazing illumination, the heart yearns to be seen and exposed under the light, appreciated for who and what it is.

Chinese medicine and other yogic traditions uphold the view of the heart as the centre of all conscious processes. With its large magnetic field, the heart, and its associated spirit, the Shen, could be compared to the sun in a solar system, while the other organs, and their associated spirit energies, would be comparable to planets, revolving around the heart's gravitational pull. If the heart is sick – on a physical, emotional or spiritual level – all other organs will be influenced. Your heart, where your Tao is 'downloaded' upon conception, is waiting for you to listen and discover it. And, like a torch in the dark, it is always there to guide you in the right direction for your soul's highest path.

ASSOCIATIONS

Spirit: Shen

Element: Fire

Yin organ: Heart

Yang organ: Small intestine

Animal: Vermilion bird

Season: Summer

Colour: Red, white and pink

Direction: South

Voice tone: Laugh

Negative emotion: Anxiety/overexcitement

Balanced emotion: Peace, contentment and joy

Physical function: Governs the health of blood vessels, circulation, and sweating

Energetic function: Keeps order. Responsible for healthy relationships to self and others; appropriate boundary setting.

Spirit function: Houses our 'soul's mandate'.
Acts as an inner compass for following our Tao.

PHYSICAL FUNCTION

The heart is a muscular organ situated in the centre of the thoracic cavity, behind and slightly left of the breastbone. About the size of a fist and enclosed in a multilayered sack of connective tissue known as the pericardium, the heart is the hardest working muscle in the human body, beating more than 100,000 times each day. Its chambers, or ventricles, serve to pump and oxygenate blood through the body through its vast network of blood vessels. Form the Western medical perspective, the heart rules the cardiovascular system and distributes blood to the body, helping to nourish cells and remove waste from them.

From the Chinese perspective, the heart is classically referred to as the 'emperor' of the entire body-mind system because, by governing the blood (cardiovascular system), it also oversees the functioning of the entire body, mind and spiritual system. Because of that, it governs all intelligent processes of the cells and, like the conductor of a symphony, ensures all organs are working in harmony. Each time the blood circulates through the heart and throughout the body, the heart takes note of what is happening and adjusts its rhythm accordingly. In addition to controlling your blood vessels, your heart regulates sweating and manifests in the complexion of your face – pale complexions or bright red complexions can indicate heart imbalances. The tongue is also closely related to the heart and is often referred to as its root – all speech impediments, such as lisps or stutters, are associated with heart pathology.

The small intestine is the paired yang (fu) organ to the heart. Physically, it is a convoluted tube that is about 2.5 centimetres (1 inch) in diameter and averages 6.4 metres (21 feet) long. It starts at the pyloric sphincter, which is the opening from the stomach, and it twists and turns through the central lower abdominal cavity before ending at the ileocecal valve, which connects to the large intestine. The functions of the small intestine in Western medicine are similar to those of Chinese medicine, in that both systems agree on its role in the reception, transformation and absorption of food content while separating the pure nutrients from waste.

ENERGETIC FUNCTION
RELATIONSHIPS AND BOUNDARY SETTING

The energetic movement of the heart, like the flame of a fire, radiates out from its centre. This radiating energy, although outward and upward moving, also has a magnetic pull and, like the sun, seeks to draw energy back in towards itself. Like the flame that reaches for the next piece of wood to burn, the heart's natural inclination is to move away from its centre to find something to latch on to. When genuine connection is achieved, this energy expands, leading to feelings of warmth, joy, gratitude and belonging.

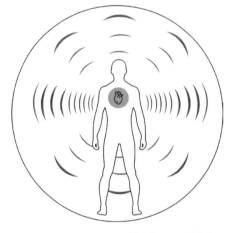

The heart's radiating energy is responsible for establishing and harmonizing our relationships: it reaches out to connect. You can see its energy in the young child who seeks your approving gaze, or in your best friend's arms as she reaches towards you for a hug. When the heart's energy is in balance, it mediates the appropriate exchange between your deep inner world and the outer word of people, animals and nature. It is the interface between your inner and outer world, and through this exchange, satisfies one of our most basic human needs: love. Without the heart's capacity to reach outwards, there would be no connection, expression or joy.

The vermilion bird, who personifies the Shen, displayers her feathers in various shades of red, resembling the vibrant flames of a fire. This bird is quick, shy and flighty. She is particular about what she eats and where she perches. You could compare the vermilion bird to your awareness that is able to travel from thought to thought, feeling to feeling, and into an imagined future or remembered past. When we enter states of meditation or sleep, the Shen resides within the heart, like the bird settling in its nest. However, when our eyes open, the Shen rises from its dwelling and settles in the eyes, preparing itself to establish connections with others. From the eyes, its light shines out, and through your speech it can express its essence – to see and be seen. After exploring, the bird eventually returns to the safety and privacy of its nest, peacefully perched in a place it can see its surroundings clearly, maintaining bright and clear-eyed awareness.

Like the little red bird, the Shen is able to intermittently venture out and return, creating a balanced rhythm of connection and retreat. Through this dynamic, the heart is able to express its authenticity, seek meaningful connections and, at the same time, maintain autonomy. It's a beautiful metaphor for the dance the heart performs – seeking both connection and retreat.

The primary relationship

The consistent return of the Shen to the home of heart helps you to establish the most important relationship of all: the relationship you have with yourself. I call this relationship the 'primary relationship' because without knowing how to relate sanely with your own mind and its many facets it is impossible to relate intimately with others. Self-hatred eventually erupts within our most intimate friends, family members and partners, mirroring back the aspects of our mind we have yet to love. Self-to-self relating is the birthplace of peace, because if you are at war with yourself you are fundamentally restless – your heart is an inhospitable place to land. Outer peace depends on inner peace.

Self-love = self-leadership

The heart, with its steady rhythmic beat, has the responsibility of maintaining order and harmony in our lives. When it is balanced, it manifests as mature self-leadership that guides us towards inner harmony, much like a conductor leads a symphony. A conductor coordinates the low and high notes, as well as the percussive elements, to create a melodic, interesting and unique composition that the audience can appreciate. Similarly, when the heart is fully in harmony, it can express itself, move and be moved by others, ultimately contributing to happiness, peace, love and joy.

While this sounds great in theory, inner harmony and self-leadership isn't always the easiest thing to achieve! If you have ever tried to meditate, or do any sort of inner work, you might have noticed that your psyche is not uni-dimensional, but rather contains a complex array of opinions and perspectives. In any given moment, you can observe the different 'voices' in your mind – the responsible part of you that manages your work schedule, the rebellious part that chimes in against the planner, the creative part that would rather be dancing, and the anxious, afraid part that just wants to stay in bed.

But you might be wondering, who exactly is relating to whom? How can 'I' establish a connection with myself if I am fragmented into various parts? Which part of 'me' is relating to the other parts of 'me'?

The 'you' that has the capacity to relate with yourself is known as the Yuan Shen, or original soul. This is the part of the Shen that is unconditioned, meaning that it is unaffected by our life circumstances. It is often described to be like sky or open space. We could also call the Yuan Shen simply 'awareness', or 'big Self' with a capital 'S'. The big Self has the ability to relate to the smaller, fragmented parts of yourself, with enough awareness to draw a consensus on what is needed based on the plethora of opinions and views within the mind. Thus, the heart gives the capacity to relate to and love all parts, like a parent to a child.

The concept of self-love is crucial to acknowledge from the beginning of your journey through the organs because it requires a certain level of compassion towards yourself as you delve into the deeper 'soul work' sections. As you unearth the darker and more embarrassing habit patterns of your mind, you will face challenges in the realm of self-love. It's easy to love the parts of yourself that are virtuous, smart and witty, but much harder to embrace your wounded, immature or emotional aspects. If you're committed to following your Tao, you must include all parts of yourself on this journey, not just those you deem 'acceptable'.

The soul work I advocate in this book isn't about pitting one part of yourself against another, but rather acknowledging the habits of your mind and gently guiding yourself towards a more authentic expression that the world can appreciate. As the poet Daniel Mead aptly puts it, 'a flower cannot be opened with a hammer'. We cannot fully open up and express ourselves if we constantly berate and criticize ourselves. A flower flourishes more under warmth and light than it ever will under force.

To be clear, loving yourself does not mean believing and acting on every thought! It also doesn't mean indulging only in 'self-care' activities, such as warm baths and pedicures, although it can sometimes manifest in that way. Similar to a loving, yet responsive parent, authentic self-love interrupts patterns that are harmful, without shaming or blaming. True self-love leads to skilful self-leadership for your highest good and for the benefit of those around you because it can consider multiple perspectives and make choices from this 'higher' vantage point. In fact, sometimes it is self-love that says 'no', or makes the hard steps you know you have to take but really don't want to.

Boundary setting

The heart's associated organs contribute to the management of our relationships by maintaining healthy boundaries. A boundary acts as a separation line between two hearts, so that the shen maintains a balance between connection and autonomy. Ironically, boundaries make relationships possible because without some degree of separation, there can be no individuality to relate to. In the framework of Chinese medicine, three organs play a role in setting boundaries: the triple warmer, the pericardium, and the small intestine.

The triple warmer, also known as the San Jiao, is a unique organ in Chinese medicine known by its function. It controls heat and fluid distribution in the body, serving as an 'invisible organ' that regulates the flow of information from the outer world to the inner world. When it comes to boundary setting, the triple warmer determines how much personal information to disclose to the public spheres and who or what is allowed into your inner world. An example could be how much you share on social media, or what your

Meanwhile, the pericardium – a fibrous sac that encloses the heart – shields it from overwhelming emotions, redirecting negative energy to the solar plexus for later processing. As the second line of defence after the triple warmer, it helps manage inner boundaries in our close relationships, determining the level of physical and emotional intimacy in any given time or situation.

Finally, the small intestine – as the yang organ counterpart to the heart – aids in discernment by distinguishing what is beneficial for personal development and by maintaining mental clarity. Like the physical role of the small intestine, which is to absorb what is pure in nutrients and what is impure, the same is true for its energetic function: it discerns what is yours and what is not. It sorts out what thoughts and intentions truly come from your heart, and which ones might have been influenced by those around you. It provides guidance on relationships that support the soul's growth and helps in untangling co-dependency in very close relationships, such as a best friend or a partner.

Expression

Another very important energetic function of the heart is its role in expression. Speech, and communicating our inner most truths to those closest to us and to the broader community, is a function of the heart. It is impossible to communicate one's truth if disconnected from it, so authentic communication and true speech first requires the Shen to be settled and one's truth to be known and felt.

As listed in the associations, the heart relates to the fire element, and the season of summer, and is represented by the blossom. During summer, shrubs, trees, flowers and bushes are in their full expression, communicating their essence through their flowering colours. Their authenticity is expressed unapologetically. This is what the heart asks of us: to communicate our truth in the way an apple tree bursts forth its apple blossom, or the way a rose patiently unfurls its crimson bud. When the heart is healthy we can know our truth and then express it. The heart animates our expression and can come out through our speech, poetry, song, or how we dress.

Joy

Genuine joy and its sister, gratitude, are expressions of the heart when it is in balance. Joy that is energetically balanced is different from the fleeting moments of happiness we may experience when we acquire a new job or car or enter a new relationship. This type of happiness, which relies on external circumstances aligning with our desires, is inconsistent and unreliable. Such happiness leads to restlessness, as we constantly try to control our lives and the external world in order to be happy. Disappointment is inevitable because life is mostly beyond our control and is constantly changing. Expecting life to always bring pleasant experiences is unrealistic, and will inevitably lead to exhaustion.

When the heart energy is balanced, we can understand that both joy and sorrow are integral parts of life, and we have the capacity to meet both. A balanced heart doesn't cling so hard to only the 'good' experiences, but can relax into the way things are.

So, what is joy if not the attainment of perfect comfort and the 'happily ever after' that the American dream promises? The joy that emanates from a balanced heart is a constant peace that arises when the heart is settled in the present moment and can find peace in whatever it meets: the smile of your partner across the room, the blossoming crocus, or the feeling of the morning sun on your cheek. This happiness is not characterized by excitement or elation, but a deep peace and contentment with what is. As written in the *Tao Te Ching*:

'Be content with what you have;
Rejoice in the way things are.
When you realize there is nothing lacking,
The whole world belongs to you.'

Stephen Mitchell,
1988 translation

Joy can also arise when you are able to act in alignment with your heart's guiding truth, making meaning out of the joy and sorrow for your development and life's winding path.

When we fully embrace our authenticity and wholeheartedly and generously contribute to the world, without worrying about the result, our heart radiates a steady, contented joy. It knows that our life has taken on the correct rhythm, and it beats in sync, not with our ego, but with the greater cadence of the universe.

SPIRITUAL FUNCTION
YOUR INNER COMPASS AND RESPONSE-ABILITY

The heart is home to the spirit of the Shen, which is both an independent spirit and the source of all of them. You can think of the Shen as pure light, and the other spirit energies as the colours that emanate from the contact of this light with the cloud. The Shen is pure consciousness, and when it comes down from heaven into a human form it divides into an array of consciousnesses expressed in the various facets of our psyche, referred to in this book as the five spirit energies.

Although each spirit rooted in each of the organs possesses its own qualities and characteristics, none of them could exist without a properly functioning heart, just as a rainbow cannot exist without the sun's light. Out of all the organs, the heart is central to our mental and spiritual health because it is what circulates consciousness through the body. The main spiritual function of the heart is self-awareness, so we can know our truths and respond appropriately.

Empty at the centre

The Chinese character for heart, *xin*, is one of the oldest in the Chinese language. It symbolizes an empty bowl with three small strokes above it. While many meanings can be pulled from this character, the empty bowl shape represents one of the primary spiritual functions of the heart: our holding capacity. The essence of the heart is the spacious background of our awareness. Through this steady witnessing presence, we can find peace and the joy already mentioned. A mind that is spacious can embrace the ebb and flow of life without being attached to a particular outcome.

The Buddha used the word *sukkha* to describe a heart that is content. Interestingly, *kha* means 'space' or the empty space at the centre of a wheel, while *su* means 'with'. During the time of the Buddha, this understanding of the world also implied a smooth ride in a cart with wheels that had the appropriate amount of space in the axle. On the other hand, *dukkha*, the term for suffering, can be translated as 'without space' and alluded to a bumpy ride in a cart with no space and friction in the axle.

The spiritual function of the heart is to provide the empty space in which the wheel of the five elements turns. Our whole life revolves around our spacious and aware heart, which can spaciously reflect or resonate and respond to the world around it.

One of the paradoxes presented by Taoist and Buddhist practices is that their teachings encourage de-accumulation, where stripping away excess leads to becoming more whole. That is, the more we strip away and return to the empty space of the heart, the more capacity we have to bear witness to the joys and sorrows of life, to see what is true, and to respond appropriately.

One of my teachers, Thanissara, gave a beautiful example of this concept during a retreat at their centre, Dhamragiri, in South Africa. It was three weeks into the retreat, and I recall struggling to meditate – gritting my teeth as I tried to implement the techniques I was learning, all the while worrying about various things that might have been going on at home. That morning, she picked up a brass singing bowl at the front of the meditation hall and rang it, creating a resonating 'wong, wong, wong' sound throughout the room. She then started to fill the bowl with random objects: a scarf, a pen, her small package of tissues, before attempting to ring it again. The sound it made was unpleasant 'tunk' that was nearly inaudible. She turned to us and said, 'Our heart is like this singing bowl. When we empty it, there is space for it to resonate with what it encounters.'

Effortless response

This process of emptying the heart, as illustrated in the singing bowl analogy, describes one of the fundamental concepts in Taoist philosophy called *wu wei*. Commonly translated as 'non-action', *wu wei* refers to the effortless way of being that leads to an easeful, healthy and meaningful life. The concept of *wu wei* presents a paradox that the more we empty ourselves of identities, harmful beliefs, presuppositions and even knowledge, the better we are equipped to know our Tao and step into its flow without wasting vital life force energy.

Wu wei is not doing nothing, kicking up your feet and watching 12 hours of Netflix while bingeing on chips! Rather, it describes the spontaneously responsive heart in its natural state: one that is clear and calm and knows how to respond. We could also call this knowing or intuition – the knowing that does not come from logic or ego, but rather the subtle pulse of life that we hear through the heart. As humans, we have this knowing capacity for the unique direction of our lives. However, if the heart is full, especially of emotionally charged beliefs, this clouds it from seeing what is true, and prevents us from responding in ways that align with our hearts.

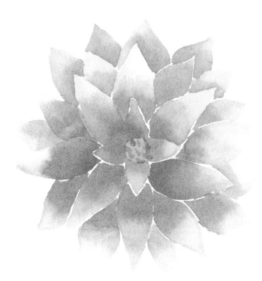

Knowing the truth

The heart is the keeper of truths: the absolute truth of our spiritual belonging and interconnection, and the relative truth of each individual life story. Following your Tao is the process of harmonizing these two universal and personal truths.

What I mean by 'truth' is a sort of resonance that the heart has with its inner and outer world. On the relative level there are as many truths as there are beings on this planet: what is true for an ant is different to what is true for your cat, or your sister or for you – there can be no absolute truth because it is always influenced by perspective. For example, for the ant crawling across your kitchen floor, it is true that your countertop is tall, but for your 6-foot-plus friend, the counter might be short. This is a simple example, but it translates to an infinite number of situations, such as relationships, careers, spirituality and how you spend your time. There is no one 'right' way to live, but there are more authentic ways to be based on what is known to be true to each individual heart. When the heart energy is balanced, it can illuminate what is true and signal direction through subtle impulses.

Many of us have been conditioned against listening to the heart's whispers because we have been heavily influenced by teachers, parents or society. Instead, we look to external sources for guidance and what is deemed 'correct'. However, by relying on external answers, we will always miss the truth. If we continue to seek answers outside ourselves, whether that be spiritual truths or others, we neglect our inner authority. This doesn't mean that we should never seek advice, read books or learn from teachers; it means that we should always consult our hearts to ensure that what we learn aligns with our own intuition.

WHERE YOU GET STUCK

The Shen leaves home

The most common and problematic issue for the heart is the scattering of energy that causes the Shen to vacate its important role as sovereign leader. In other words, the mind leaves the body. Any level of shock, trauma or overwhelm can cause the vermilion bird to flee from its home. This includes big traumas, such as a car accident or losing a loved one suddenly, or can be smaller instances, such as a stern email from our boss or even when a friend jumps out playfully from round a corner.

In cases of extreme shock or trauma, the Shen leaves completely, and there can be a feeling of being totally outside of the body, a perception that the world is not real, and a confused sense of identity, including long-term amnesia of certain events. Since the heart is where consciousness resides, and acts as the keeper of long-term memory and lasting sense of identity, it makes sense that these abilities are lost when shocked or traumatized. In Western psychological terms, this is called 'dissociation' and is often reserved as a symptom for those in extreme shock or recovering from trauma.

From a medical qigong perspective, extreme trauma can fracture a part of the Shen and lock it away in the past. That is, there is a part of us that never returns after a major trauma, mirroring the sayings, 'I lost a part of myself that day' or 'I was never the same after that'. Part of the healing work for the heart is recovering aspects of the Shen that were lost during traumatic events. This can take time and usually requires support from a qualified therapist or alternative practitioner.

Overwhelm anxiety

As you learned in the previous section, the strength of the heart is defined by having space. The Shen spirit can flee simply because there isn't any space for it, perhaps because of constant exposure to media, excessive workload and overwhelming situations, which leave us in a state of chronic anxiety. While anxiety is also connected to the kidneys, the subtle restlessness and constant inability to fully find peace in the present moment are associated with the heart, and the little red birds of the Shen who cannot find rest.

Nervous laughter

Another dissociative tendency characterized by heart imbalance is incongruent emotion – laughing at something serious or traumatic, or smiling when recalling a painful memory. The voice tone of the heart is a laugh – and nervous laughter is a sign that the Shen isn't home to fully witness the pain of an event and can even be a way to further avoid that emotional pain.

Excitement/elation

Negative shock is one way that will cause the spirit to flee, but the spirit can also become overwhelmed by positive experiences. As you have learned, joy is a deeply grounded experience that occurs when the heart is open, connected and at peace, and when there is rhythm and harmony in one's life. Excitement, which is often confused with joy in Western culture, is classified in Chinese medicine as a negative emotion that disrupts the mind. This is because it causes the spirit to leave the heart, similar to how shock or trauma would, leading to similar tendencies of dissociation. The word 'excitement' itself comes from the Latin word *excitare*, which means to rouse, call out or stir up. The prefix 'ex-' (as in 'exit') even implies that there is a movement of one's mind in an outward direction.

Unfortunately, modernity promotes extreme states of 'happiness'. The result is that many of us have developed a tendency for constant stimulation, which has become a habit and addiction. The hunger for excitement keeps the heart in a restless state, leading to chronic detachment and a disconnection from our bodies and our souls.

Falling in love

A classic example of excitation causing an imbalance of heart energy is falling in love. Falling in love happens when the Shen recognizes the inherent perfection of its own soul within the other, like a mirror. When you fall in love, you do not see the whole person, with their flaws and idiosyncrasies, but rather your Shen sees only the light in the other's Shen shining back. Like a deer in headlights, you are pulled into the light, falling into the other with your whole heart.

In the process of seeing and being seen, love spurs overwhelming feelings of joy, which causes the heart to beat faster and Shen to fly up to the heaven and the qi to scatter. With your Shen not at home in the heart, your life might take on a state of disorder and feel as though your 'head is in the clouds'. In this state, it is common to abandon other facets of your life that were important to you before your new love interest. In extreme cases, romantic love might lead you to believe that you lover is what completes you, and the line between what is 'me' and what is 'you' becomes blurred. This is why you might make decisions you will regret later when 'under the influence' of love. You might look back after waking up from the spell of love and say to yourself, 'What was I thinking?'

I am not saying to deny the experience of falling in love, but to remember that if the Shen is gone, all other organs and their intelligences will be affected and access to responsive self-leadership is impaired. In these sorts of states of excitation, we might say something we don't mean or make a decision that is opposite to our deepest values.

Sleep disturbances and mood swings

There are other consequences of an excited heart, including insomnia and dream-disturbed sleep. Not sleeping well will impact our qi and deplete it, also impacting the functioning of our brain and our mood. In addition, when the Shen departs from the body, a significant amount of our vital energy (qi) also leaves. As a result, excitement drains our energy, which is why it is often followed by a feeling of exhaustion. A minor case of this can be observed in the build-up to exciting events, such as a wedding or graduation. There is a great deal of excitement leading up to the event and during it, but afterwards, there is a drop in our mood. Excitement can also happen when we are overstimulated at a shopping mall – perhaps we are with a group of friends and see something that we want that promises us a better life. In this state of excitement, we might impulsively buy things we can't afford and, upon coming down off our high, regret our purchases. It is important to remember that Taoism emphasizes the importance of balance rather than extremes. Even though excitement can feel positive, it is an intense emotion that drains us, like the effects of a hangover. In extreme cases, this can manifest as extreme shifts between elation and depression, which Western psychiatrists would refer to as a manic-depressive episode or bipolar disorder.

Self-doubt

Self-doubt arises when the inner authority of the heart is questioned or ignored. The longer we ignore the subtle impulses of the Shen, the less we hear them, and the more we step out of touch with the natural rhythm of our life. While certain obligations make it impossible to follow every impulse our heart has, following none of them, especially ones that are deeply important to us, is detrimental for our soul's development and can lead to deep regret. Palliative care nurse Bronnie Ware writes in her international bestselling memoir, *The Top Five Regrets of the Dying*, that the number one regret of her palliative patients was 'I wish I'd had the courage to live a life true to myself, not the life others expected of me.'

So why does doubt happen? Why do we ignore our inner authority? While the heart is our compass, it also yearns to connect. If we do not feel a deep connection with ourselves and the natural world, we compromise our true selves to fit in with others, even if that connection is shallow and obstructs our personal growth.

While friends, family or the internet might have good advice about what direction you should take in your life, it is not your direction. In relying on others to guide you, or following along the path of societal 'shoulds' you risk dimming the light of your Shen and stunting the growth of who you are naturally meant to be. Like binding the blossoming of a flower, this is detrimental to your soul's development. It also robs others of the gift that we are meant to shine.

Symptoms of imbalance

Take a look at the symptoms opposite, which can arise when the heart and small intestine energies are thrown off. If you notice any of these as themes in your life, especially if you experience one symptom in each category, it might indicate your heart and the fire phase needs some love!

PHYSICAL

* cardiovascular disease
* palpitations
* insomnia
* sweaty palms
* inflammation (excess heat)
* sluggish digestion (deficient heat)
* bright red or pale facial complexion

ENERGETIC

* nightmares/dream disturbed sleep
* anxiety
* restlessness
* hyperactivity or mania
* poor boundaries
* a closed-off heart
* scattered attention, 'head in the clouds'
* lack of joy
* feeling disconnected from self and others
* inappropriate laughter

SPIRITUAL

* inability to self-reflect
* confusion about your life path
* poor self-leadership
* self-doubt
* relying on external validation to discern what is right for you
* inability to discern what is 'true' versus what is 'false'

SOUL WORK
FROM CHAOS TO CLARITY

The soul work for the heart is an invitation to create more space in your life for the Shen to settle back into the body. Once the Shen is home, you are clear about your life's direction, can nurture healthy relationships and are present for the joy the present moment offers.

Physical Soul Work

Because the heart relates to the fire element, physical issues related to the heart can show up as excess or deficient heat in the body. The summer season is a time when the fire element can be thrown off, and we can become too hot. Making sure you are getting enough fluids and monitoring your intake of spicy and high-fat foods can help lower overall heat.

To nourish your physical heart, including moderate cardiovascular exercise, such as brisk walking, running, or cycling, in your weekly routine can help the physical organ stay strong. It is also important to include physical activities that lower mental stress, such as yoga, qigong or deep breathing, which will all help settle the rising and scattering qi that can lead to excess heat and physical heart issues, such as arrhythmia and hypertension.

To nourish the small intestine, it is important you are eating foods that your body can digest and absorb so that you are getting the appropriate nutrients and vitamins. Parasitic infections can be hard on the small intestine, and will also prevent you from absorbing the proper nutrients you need. If you have travelled or live in a country where parasite infections are common, it might be good idea to seek support from a naturopath or other healthcare practitioner who can assess and help treat these infections.

The heart and small intestine organ pair relate to the bitter taste and the colour red, so including bitter foods in your diet, such as dandelion greens, celery, coffee (in moderation), cacao, tea and parsley, and red foods such as watermelon, strawberries and tomatoes, can help to nourish these organs.

When the heart energy is balanced, we can
understand that both joy
and sorrow are integral parts of life,
and we have the capacity to meet both.

A balanced heart doesn't cling so hard
to only the 'good' experiences
but can relax into the way things are.

EXERCISE
BRINGING DOWN THE HEAVENS

This simple qigong practice encourages the downward flow of energy that can help calm any physical agitation of the heart. You can practise this anytime, anywhere, and it takes less than five minutes to complete. If you find you have a lot of stress, you could even do this at work by taking a short break several times per day.

1 Begin by standing with your feet shoulder-distance apart, knees slightly bent, shoulders relaxed and your tailbone down. Imagine your feet have roots growing out of them, or that you are standing in mud up to your ankles. Take a few deep breaths and relax as you stand firmly.

2 Imagine your hands are like magnets. As you inhale, reach your arms up and imagine gathering a golden light. This light carries the energy of contentment, peace and grounded presence. You can also imagine that it carries the energy of your Shen – as though you are re-gathering all parts of yourself home.

3 Exhale, and turn your hands to face the earth. Continue to exhale as you descend the hands down the front of the body, imagining the light running from the crown of the head, down the forehead, face, neck, chest and all the way down the entire front line of the body to the toes. Imagine this light is illuminating every cell with peaceful presence.

4 Complete a second round of the previous two movements, but this time, imagine the light illuminating the back line of the body, rinsing like a golden oil from the back of the head to the heels.

5 On the third and final round, imagine the light entering through the crown of the head, illuminating the brain, and flowing down the centre of the body, filling all the organs, rinsing down the centre of each leg bone, all the way down into the feet and into the earth.

6 After the three rounds of bringing the energy down, notice how you feel.

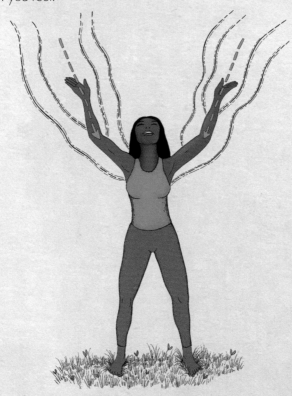

Energetic Soul Work

To nourish your heart on an energetic level, it is essential to develop healthy relationships with yourself, others and nature. Developing a relationship with yourself might be the hardest of all, so please do not panic if you find it difficult! To start this process, spending some quiet time each day with yourself (perhaps practising the exercises in this section) can be an initiation into this relationship. On the days you cannot find the time to be alone, you could simply notice how you relate to the various 'parts' of your mind throughout a workday. If you notice your inner dialogue is harsh or aggressive, is it possible to speak to yourself the way you would speak to a friend or family member? You could even just interrupt that critical voice and take a breath. What does the critical voice need to feel safe and connected? If you are a visual person, you could imagine these parts, or 'voices', in your mind, to be friends or family members gathered around a fire, each with their own viewpoint and longing to be happy. Without needing to 'love' any of these inner parts, can you just give space for them to be and to hear their perspective? This exercise may help the seed of self-warmth and connection take root in your heart.

Nurturing relationships with other people, animals and places in nature where you feel that you can safely be yourself and express yourself is essential for the Shen to shine. Even if you are an introverted person, the Shen cannot fully blossom in isolation, because it longs to be seen and to express itself. This could be as simple as phoning a friend or attending a social gathering. On the flip side, the soul work for the heart could also mean avoiding or ending relationships and situations that diminish your sense of self and agitate the mind.

Choosing the right relationships and the appropriate levels of connection is especially important for our heart health. Remember that boundaries include both what comes and goes from your heart. You might notice yourself over-sharing or developing intimacy in relationships too quickly. Or, perhaps, you notice that your heart is guarded and you don't let anyone in. Are your boundaries too rigid or too loose? Because our ability to set and maintain boundaries is injured by past interpersonal relationships, talking with a therapist about boundary violations and trust issues can be especially helpful, as interpersonal wounds are only healed through interpersonal exchanges.

In addition to fostering relationships, joy nourishes the heart and is essential for the soul's development, and is an emotion that can be trained. Psychologist Rick Hanson collected numerous neurological studies in his book *Hardwiring Happiness* that suggest that positive experiences take longer for the mind to register compared to negative ones. We often overlook the numerous positive moments that occur each day because we're not attentive. These moments could be as simple as savouring your morning coffee or sharing a smile with a colleague.

So, rather than actively seeking out more things that make you happy, take the time to fully appreciate the joy you've already experienced. I make it a habit with my partner to discuss our gratitude before we take our first bite of dinner, and to talk about our favourite parts of the day before bed. You can easily incorporate this into your family routine or, if you live alone, try journalling or reflecting on enjoyable moments as you fall asleep, letting your imagination relive them.

EXERCISE
HEART BREATHING PART 1: CREATING SPACE

This part of the exercise creates more space in your heart to be in relationship with whatever arises, helping to increase patience and stability of mind. The practice is a variation of 'heart breathing', as taught by the HeartMath institute. It utilizes two acupressure points, one at the front of the chest, known as the Sea of Tranquility, and one at the back known as the Spirit Path. Bringing your attention to your breath and these points is short, effective and can be practised almost anywhere and anytime!

1 Take a moment to sit comfortably. Relax the root of your tongue, your jaw and face. Connect to your heart as you bring both your hands over or on the Sea of Tranquility point.

2 If you are comfortable to do so, close your eyes and feel the Shen settle from your eyes down to your heart. Notice your breath, and take a few deeper ones so you can really get in touch with it, feeling the pressure of your hands on that point.

3 Relax your hands away from your body and imagine your heart has two noses, one at the front of the chest along the Sea of Tranquility and one on the back, around the Spirit Path.

4 Imagine breathing in through the front nose of the heart, and out the back nose; then in through the back and out the front. If possible, extend the breath to a slow count of five in, and a slow count of five out. Breathe into the heart through the front, and out the back, in the back, and out the front.

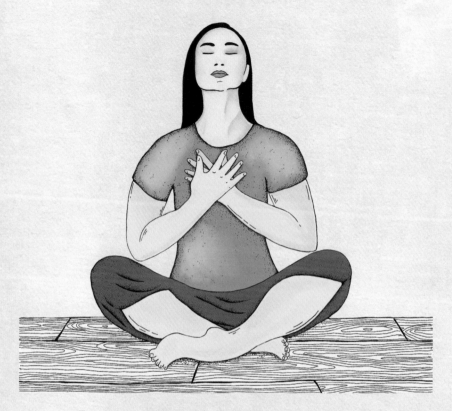

Feel how pendulating the breath creates more space around the heart – like opening two windows on either side of a room to create a cross breeze. There is nothing to think about other than this breath. Repeat for between five and nine cycles.

5 After a few rounds of moving the breath to the front and to the back of the heart, sense the heart and its empty centre. Rest your attention there, and breathe quietly and naturally. Enjoy the space to just be, noticing any messages that the heart has for you.

EXERCISE
HEART BREATHING PART 2: HEART SMILING

This part of the exercise is a way you can 'soak in' the joy and help embody the practice of gratitude more fully.

1 Bring to mind someone or something that makes you smile. It could be anything – a pet, a person, something happy that happened, or even something funny. Preferably, visualize that thing until it puts a physical smile to your face.

2 Now, let that image in your mind fade, but keep the feeling behind it. Breathe in the energy of that smile into both the front and back gates of your heart and, as you exhale, feel that joy filling the heart like water into a bathtub.

3 Repeat this nine times, or until you feel your heart expand and radiate in a balanced and peaceful way.

Spiritual Soul Work

On a spiritual level, the soul work for the heart involves creating enough space in your life for your Shen to settle in its nest. Because the heart is destabilized, mainly by overstimulation and overwhelm, I recommend taking time each day to just be. These moments can take the form of a peaceful walk, driving alone to the grocery store, or simply spending five minutes to practise one of the exercises in this book. Incorporating consistent meditation into your routine can be a powerful way to settle the Shen, and, if you don't already practise meditation, I highly recommend starting.

Silence, in particular, holds a special significance in nourishing the Shen, because it encourages the energy typically used for talking and engaging with the outside world to settle within the heart. Personally, I take extended time in my life for silence, such as a silent retreat or silent time by myself in nature daily. A short daily period of silence, such as five minutes, is more effective in the long run than an hour-long period once a week. The more frequently you check in with yourself, the greater the opportunity for your Shen to find its home and for you to align with your own truth instead of being influenced solely by external factors. What you might find, is that the time investment of taking quiet time to check in with yourself will be well worth it, as your life will take on more order and rhythm as your Shen begins to guide your life.

In addition to taking time to 'be', the soul work for the heart entails listening to your own truths and, eventually, mustering up the courage to defend those truths through your words and actions. This involves the small intestine's gift of discerning what is true for you, and what is not. Over time, we learn to cultivate the skill of discerning what truly resonates with our hearts, rather than solely relying on our rational thinking minds. This process allows us to develop a deeper connection with our authentic selves.

EXERCISE
HEART READING: WHAT DOES A 'YES' FEEL LIKE?

I have described the heart in this chapter as the leader, the guiding compass, or as 'the only book worth reading'. So, how do you 'read the heart'? This exercise will help acquaint you with these subtle feelings and translate them into knowing.

1 Begin by practising a few rounds of heart breathing (see pages 62–4).

2 Then, deliberately tell your heart a lie, something that isn't true. For example, 'My name is Fred', or 'I love baseball'. Notice what happens when you tell the heart a lie. What sort of sensations does the heart produce? Does the lie resonate with the heart? If not, what does the heart do in response to this untruth?

3 Next, deliberately tell your heart something you know to be true. For example, if you are a mother, say something like, 'I love my daughter', or you can say out loud what your name is or the place you live. Notice what the heart does in response to something true.

4 Go back and forth between the lie and the truth, and feel the difference between the sensations of the heart. You might notice that the truth carries more of a resonance than the lie. Maybe there is a warmth, or a trembling or a refined expansion.

This simple practice can be used to return to your inner authority when faced with a large question, such as 'Should I take that new job?' or 'Would this relationship be good for me?' It can also be practised with small questions, such as 'Should I go to the party tonight?' The heart is always expanding and contracting, picking up on information to direct our life's path. 'Yes or no' questions are usually most effective for this exercise, but you can use it for questions that are more open, and meditate on the innumerable feelings that the heart produces when imagining possible life directions. It can also be used to determine what your boundaries are within a relationship, and when you need to assert a 'no' to protect the heart and its authority.

I recommend first practising this with small questions, such as 'Should I go to the party tonight?', or even consulting your heart on what route you should take when driving to work. What happens when you listen to the heart's intuition? What happens when you don't?

If you feel disconnected from your heart and don't get any feeling when asking questions, you can also listen in to the small intestine, the heart's yang counterpart in the centre of the abdomen. For some, 'gut' impulses are reflective of their heart's truths.

CHAPTER 2
Dare to Dream

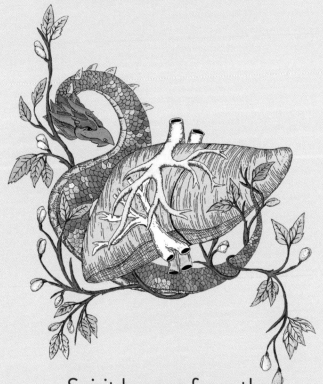

Spirit lessons from the
liver and gallbladder

'Hope is the only bee that makes
honey without flowers.'

Robert Green

I walk through one of the last remaining old-growth temperate rainforests on the west coast of Vancouver Island, my feet soaked from puddles of spring rain. Life thrives in every season under this canopy, but today the scene appears more vibrant – the forest floor a tapestry of bright green ferns, mosses and fungi reflected in the morning sun. Eventually, I approach an ancient cedar giant, whose presence forces me to pause. As I move to her side, I see that her roots open into a cavern. I take my backpack off and squeeze between the roots and stand inside the centre. An immediate feeling of calm and reverence enters my heart. Safe in this secluded enclave, far from the reaches of modernity, I feel as though I have entered a temple. I look up in awe of the innards of her bark – the twist and turns of her wood, veins outlining the creative manoeuvres she has made over centuries in search of nutrients, to reach the light and to grow. I can feel her energy saying, 'Up we go, no matter what, I will become!'. I wonder if, as a seedling, this tree ever dreamt it was possible to reach this height against all odds. I wonder if she ever hoped that, in all her efforts, she would give so much back to the land and to the creatures she now houses, shades and feeds. As I stand in this tree, I feel the impossible as a reality. The seed that was once a delicate sprout, fighting to make her way through the rocks, is now as tall as a skyscraper, and so wide I can barely reach round her perimeter.

Trees embody the qualities of determination, boldness, passion for growth and endless generosity. Their becoming benefits millions of life forms, including bacteria, insects, fungi, animals, birds, and our atmosphere. Like the wood phase, the rising sun and its associated season of spring, the liver energy is our inner tree: thrusting up towards new horizons, pushing us in a 'ready or not' way towards growth. The wood phase inside you is held in your liver and gallbladder organs and is what allows you to grow and expand towards new horizons so that you can share your gifts with the world.

The spirit animal of the liver is the green dragon, who reminds us of the buoyancy of imagination, the authority of creativity and dreams. He is the driving force that brings what is invisible (our hopes, plans and visions) to light, and aids in our decision making. The power of the green dragon lends us our capacity to take a stand against injustices and defend our personal truth. He is a benevolent protector that rises for the possibility of a brighter future.

When out of balance, the liver, gallbladder and the wood element can express as anger and frustration, and as ceaseless striving that leaves us exhausted; but when in harmony, offers the faculties of fierce compassion and the gumption it takes to leap into new territory. Like the cedar tree, the liver wants us to grow our whole life – stagnation is its enemy, movement is its motif. It won't rest until the colours of its dream start to bleed from the edges of your imagination into the reality of your notebook. The liver is what inspires us to dream of a new possibility, regardless of the circumstances we find ourselves in.

ASSOCIATIONS

Spirit: Hun

Element: Wood

Yin organ: Liver

Yang organ: Gallbladder

Animal: Green dragon

Season: Spring

Colour: Green

Direction: East

Voice tone: Shout

Sense: Sight

Negative emotion: Anger, resentment, frustration, shame, guilt, depression and hopelessness

Balanced emotion: Compassion

Physical function: Governs the smooth flow of qi; stores the blood; governs the health of the eyes, small muscles and tendons

Energetic function: Emotional regulation, fierce caring, motivation to act

Spirit function: Dreams and visions, plans and decision making

PHYSICAL FUNCTION
THE FLOW OF BLOOD AND QI

On a physical level, the liver is the largest organ within the body and sits underneath the ribcage on the right side. It comprises about two percent of your body weight, weighing an average of 1.3 kilograms (3 pounds), and is about the size of an American football. From the Western medical perspective, it supports an array of different functions in the body, including metabolism, immunity, digestion, detoxification and vitamin storage.

From the Chinese energetic perspective, the liver is responsible for the smooth movement of blood and qi. When we are physically active, the liver facilitates the flow of blood from itself into the muscles and tendons, promoting their health and flexibility. Just like its associated season, spring, and the wood phase that pushes new growth up from the soil, the liver pushes our blood towards areas that require nourishment, renewing blood flow and energy circulation. Through the movement of blood and qi, the liver manages the health of our small muscles and tendons, our nails and the health of our eyes. All problems relating to vision have their root in liver health. The liver is also responsible for detoxification, ridding the body and blood of harmful waste and toxins. Because of its relationship to blood, the liver is closely related to the proper functioning of the uterus, menstruation and breast health. Premenstrual symptoms, irregular menstruation and other gynaecological issues are often closely associated with the liver energy.

The main point to remember about the physical function of the liver is that it prevents energy stagnation. When qi is stagnant, it leads to blockages in the energy channels, which impacts other organ systems as well. Some chronic symptoms of liver qi stagnation are migraines, cysts, tumours and even some cancers. While there are various factors involved in these symptoms, the smooth and even flow of qi holds paramount importance in maintaining good health. As the Chinese medicine saying goes, 'If there is pain, there is no free flow; if there is free flow, there is no pain.'

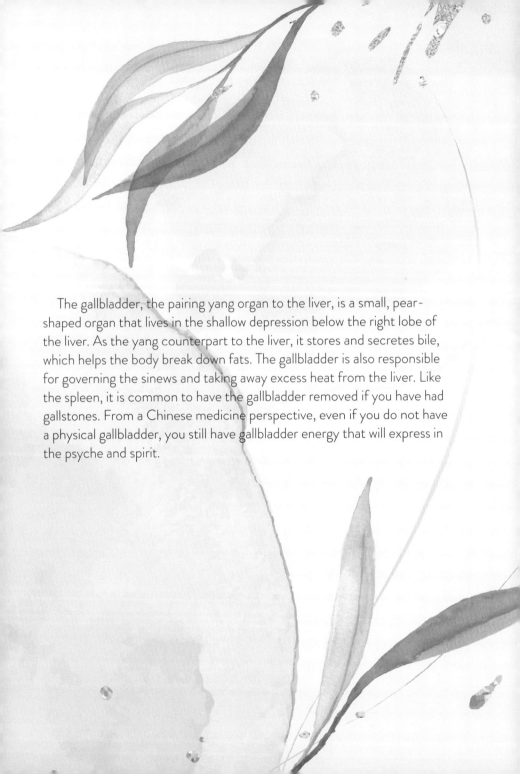

The gallbladder, the pairing yang organ to the liver, is a small, pear-shaped organ that lives in the shallow depression below the right lobe of the liver. As the yang counterpart to the liver, it stores and secretes bile, which helps the body break down fats. The gallbladder is also responsible for governing the sinews and taking away excess heat from the liver. Like the spleen, it is common to have the gallbladder removed if you have had gallstones. From a Chinese medicine perspective, even if you do not have a physical gallbladder, you still have gallbladder energy that will express in the psyche and spirit.

ENERGETIC FUNCTION
EMOTIONAL REGULATION AND COMPASSION

The energetic function of the liver mirrors its physical function in its emphasis on movement and flow. The liver pushes upwards. Like a sprouting weed in spring that pushes up through a cement crack against all odds, the liver faithfully defends its becoming. Remember that all organs are in communication with the Shen, and are of service to your Tao. When out of balance, this upward, pushing energy loses touch with the heart and can manifest as anger and rage, but when in balance, it gives you the energy to push forward towards your goals, set appropriate boundaries and make essential decisions that are of service to your life's path. This pushing energy demands space for the heart's values and is fearless in its need to grow into its full expression.

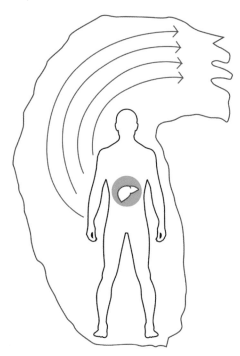

The liver energy is what lives behind the question 'What's next?'. It is growth-oriented, at times competitive, and is always striving to improve. It is the energy behind every aspiration, daydream and crazy idea. Like the powerful green dragon who rises from earth to heaven, bringing about transformation and renewal, the liver urges us forward to prevent our life from stagnating. The Chinese dragon is flexible, fast, agile and, at times, ferocious. He is an embodiment of the yang movement of our soul, and knows that if the movement stops, we will be sucked down by the entropic force of an old story. The liver cares about the world and wants to write a new story, one that is fresh and alive with the Shen's authenticity and light.

Emotional regulation

On an energetic level, one of the main functions of the liver is to regulate our emotions. Emotions are qi, and they need to move. The term 'emotion' literally means 'to move'. Since the liver is responsible for facilitating the smooth movement of qi, when someone has balanced liver energy, they generally have an even temperament, allowing their emotions to move without getting excessively attached to them or suppressing them.

Our emotional temperament is impacted by the physical state of the liver. If there is liver qi stagnation, it will often lead to frustration and irritability or an uneven temperament. For instance, during a woman's menstrual cycle, the body's effort to move the blood puts strain on the liver, disrupting the flow of energy and causing irritability and mood changes. Another example is excessive alcohol consumption, which can induce anger due to the liver being affected and compromising qi flow.

Emotional regulation also involves the spiritual aspect of the liver, and the proper functioning of the liver spirit known as the Hun. The Hun is our conscience. It has the ability to temper our more primitive responses that arise from the body's various energetic waves. The Hun helps us establish our moral standards and discern right from wrong, and presses the 'pause' button before we react.

From the Western perspective, the energetic function of both the liver and the heart can be compared to the frontal lobes of our brain, which are related to our morality and higher cognitive processes of meta cognition, altruism and compassion. This part of our mind is like the inner parent that can help us self-regulate and calm the more childish parts of ourselves that are scared, anxious or rebellious. Both the liver and the heart are related to this self-regulatory process. However, the liver, and its associated spirit the Hun, is the active participatory agent – it is the firm voice in your head that guides you away from making decisions that lead to harm or that you will regret later. Through the conscience, the liver helps us stay in alignment with the heart's authority, and course-corrects when we go against what is true in our heart. Psychologically, someone with healthy liver energy is able to live in accordance with their moral standards while also allowing their emotions to flow, and can feel their feelings without being taken over by them.

The Hun also helps to regulate our emotions through self-compassion. The self-compassion of the liver, however, is more yang (active) then the self-love of the heart, which is more soothing. The self-compassion of the liver is a caring force that can respond when needed to any action to prevent emotional upheaval from continuing.

Fierce caring

A tree strives to grow, not just for its own benefit, but to contribute to the ecosystem. Trees enable land creatures to breathe by exchanging carbon dioxide with oxygen, prevent soil erosion and mitigate the impact of windstorms. Moreover, they demonstrate altruism within their own community. Studies have revealed that trees communicate through fungal networks, and they share nutrients with each other when injured or with their young saplings, ensuring the survival of felled trees as 'living stumps'.

The same is true for the wood phase in your body. When guided by the light of the Shen (your awareness), the energy behind the liver's 'push' is caring. It is a force that will stand up against those who are powerless and fights for growth to benefit the collective. The liver is known to be associated with anger, which gets a bad reputation since it can lead to violence and harm. Although anger can be a toxic emotion when it is untethered to the heart, when it is worked with intentionally, its energy is absolutely essential for the preservation of life and helps us to stand up for what we care about.

For example, the cedar tree I described in this chapter's opening owes its existence to the thousands of protesters who rallied against the logging industry in the early nineties. Determined to save the old-growth forest on Meares Island (on Vancouver Island's west coast), over 800 peaceful protesters were arrested for blocking roads and safeguarding trees that were over 1,500 years old. The beauty and biodiversity I experienced in the forest that day would have been clear-cut for furniture, lumber, and firewood if it wasn't for the spirit of the liver and gallbladder! While anger can be toxic, it also helps us to set boundaries around what we care about. It safeguards our perception of right and wrong and can serve as a motivational force for change. It compels us to envision new possibilities and embark on transformative journeys that might at the time require resistance and a tremendous amount of force.

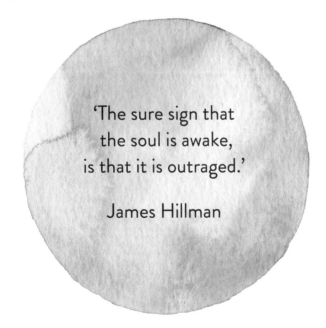

'The sure sign that
the soul is awake,
is that it is outraged.'

James Hillman

SPIRITUAL FUNCTION
DREAMS, IMAGINATION AND PLANS

While the energy of the liver provides the force for growth, the spirit of the liver guides and directs that growth through visions, imaginations and dreams.

As you have learned, the Hun is the spirit of the liver and is our conscience. Like the Shen, the Hun is a yang spirit from heaven, helping to direct our life from a conscious level. The main difference between the two is that our Shen holds the Tao while the Hun dreams up possibilities of how that Tao will exist on the material plane. The Shen, although holding the 'ultimate truth', only points in a general direction through impulse and sudden insights of 'Yes!' or 'No!'. It does not offer details of how to move in that direction. It is the spirit of the liver, the Hun, that starts to take those insights and break them down into something more tangible: a dream, a vision, a plan and, eventually, a first step.

Just as the liver maintains the physical health of our eyes and sight, on a spiritual level it gifts us our internal vision through our dreams and imagination. It is said that when we dream, both in the day through our active imagination and in the night through sleep, the Hun soul flies up into heaven, providing us with the creativity we need to enact the Shen's instructions. In other words, the Hun provides us with the spiritual eye – to see where we are going next and to make sure it is in line with the heart's deepest truths.

The liver also provides us with creative eyes, the ones that can see and appreciate beauty. Any time you participate in a creative endeavour, you are exercising your inner vision and the spirit of your liver. The liver helps you to see the potential for beauty where there is none, and reminds you that renewal is always possible.

Decision-making

While the spirit of the liver envisions future possibilities, painting the plan in our mind's eye, the gallbladder on a spiritual level takes those dreams and sketches out a detailed plan, with a timeline, an agenda and actionable steps.

The gallbladder holds and then releases the concentrated energy needed to 'pull the trigger' on big decisions: the phone call to buy the house or take the job, or click the button to sign up for the marathon. Just like the concentrated bile it stores and releases at exactly the right time, the gallbladder releases its bout of bravery and boldness to step into new territory. Timidity and inability to make decisions are a result of this energy being hindered or undernourished. We need to have the 'gall' to take risks, to step outside of our comfort zone, in order to grow.

The gallbladder energy is also used on smaller decisions, such as what peanut butter to buy at the grocery store or what route to take on the way to work. Again, it is absolutely essential that our decisions be tethered to the Shen and tempered by our conscience and Hun; otherwise, these decisions can be impulsive and guide us further away from our Tao, rather than closer to it.

The imagination

The imagination is one of the most important human capacities that the Hun spirit offers us, because it creates tension between what is and what isn't possible. This tension generates the forward momentum for growth, and the liver energy with its 'pushing force' helps us ride the wave of that tension. All ideas and moral vision depend on imagination. The symphony, the movie you saw last weekend, the bridge you drove across to get to work, every piece of furniture that is in your living room – all of these things you enjoy had to exist once solely in someone's imagination. The imagination is your capacity to see without eyes, to hear without ears – and to project a new reality into the future. It provides us with the capacity to hope, and prevents us from slipping into despair.

There is a story that exemplifies the power of imagination, told of the celebrated French poet Robert Desnos in World War II by Norman Fischer in his book *The World Could Be Otherwise*. Desnos was of Jewish descent, and part of the French resistance movement against the Nazi party; he was eventually captured and sent to a concentration camp. One day, the prisoners in his camp were loaded on to a flatbed truck to be transported from their barracks to the gas chambers. As they disembarked, the atmosphere was suffocatingly sad – no one said a word, not even the guards, who could sense the energy of the grim occasion. As the prisoners began to shuffle forward, heading towards the next truck that would lead them to their inevitable fate, Desnos broke away from the line and seized the hand of the woman in front of him. With a renewed sense of animation, he started to examine her palm and do a palm reading, the way a fortune-teller would. 'You will live a long life... and have many grandchildren, and abundant joy!,' he exclaimed loudly, so the other prisoners and guards could hear.

The spark Desnos ignited drew the attention of someone nearby, who promptly offered his palm for inspection. With each palm thrust towards him, Desnos prophesied a similarly optimistic future – long and joyous lives filled with happiness and success. The other prisoners, emboldened by these glimpses of hope, eagerly extended their palms to Desnos. Their collective despair momentarily lifted, replaced by the possibility, smiling and laughing.

The mood was infectious to the guards, who were confused and disorientated. The prisoners, now laughing and celebrating their futures, became not just numbered prisoners but humans with imagined and hopeful futures. Desnos had shifted the reality of everyone in the group, so much so that the guards did not follow through with their executions. Imagination saved the lives of Desnos and his fellow inmates that day.

Not only is the imagination a powerful creative force for the external world, but it is always a powerful creative force for the growth of our inner world. We can actively use our imagination to heal past traumas, enquire into our outdated patterns and engage in dialogue with dream characters or certain aspects of our psyche that require love and care. In qigong therapy, imagination is extensively utilized in various practices, prescription exercises and treatments because it helps direct energy flow. We know imagination can cause physiological responses: if you think about the food you really want to have, it might make you hungry! Or imagining erotic images can arouse your body. Or when you bring to mind someone you really love, you might feel this physically as a heart opening. For centuries, yogis from many cultures and traditions have used this faculty of imagination to direct their inner life towards greater expansion and wellbeing.

Imagination provides us with another very important ability, and that is the capability to be compassionate. Compassion, which means 'to suffer with', requires us to empathize and share the suffering of others. How can we understand and empathize with others if we don't use our imagination? When we imagine being someone else, especially someone experiencing pain, compassion naturally arises. Compassion then leads us to envision new and improved ways of existing in the world, which can alleviate the suffering of others and ultimately benefit everyone. Imagination fuels compassionate feeling and movement into compassionate action.

'Yes: I am a dreamer.
For a dreamer is one who can only find his way by moonlight, and his punishment is that he sees the dawn before the rest of the world.'

Oscar Wilde, *The Critic As Artist* (1891)

WHERE YOU GET STUCK
BLINDED BY ANGER

Anger is a powerful energy that can be harnessed for justice, but it can also lead to acting or speaking in ways we regret and which are out of alignment with our heart's deepest values. The expression 'I lost my temper' implies that anger is something that can get away from us or take us over. Because it is such a strong energy, anger can be a slippery slope that can lead to violence towards yourself or another. It can also become an ingrained personality trait, leading people to become bitter, mistrusting and unkind. If your energy is being consumed by anger, it can be really exhausting. If you are deeply engaged in social justice work, it is important to guard against anger consuming your mind, which can shadow the joy that also exists in life.

Where the energy of anger goes wrong is when we are blinded by it. Remember, the Shen and the Hun rest in our eyes, directing actions of body, speech and mind that align with what we value most. When we are in a state of rage, liver energy rises from the inner groin and out of the eyes, clouding our vision and the ability to see any perspective other than that of our anger. The imaginative capacities of the Hun are impaired, limiting our compassion and the wisdom of our response.

Anger is merely an expression of energy, and a strong defence mechanism that is usually pointing to an unmet need within us or someone else. Once we can calm our emotions down enough to be in relationship with our anger, we are no longer angry but are seeing our anger as an upward moving energy that is there to protect, relate to and express in a healthy way. We get stuck when we become our anger and fully embody it, rather than relate to it.

Supressing anger

Anger is toxic when expressed outwardly, but can be equally toxic when it is repressed. The rising energy of anger is like a dragon flying out of a cave: it is a strong force! Supressing that energy is like chaining the dragon down and closing in the cave walls. The supressed anger from the initial event doesn't ever go away – rather, it sits and festers in the body. The dragon within you grows more angry, impatient and restless. If it isn't released, this will lead to blood stagnation and other energetic imbalances, and even cause the body to attack itself.

One of the most common issues of anger suppression I have seen in the qigong clinic are women with endometriosis, tumours of the ovaries or cervix and other gynaecological issues. Perhaps one of the reasons why this issue is more common is because women have been taught to supress anger and told that anger isn't pretty or nice, or wanted. Supressing anger will eventually lead to blood stagnation, which can lead to physical complications in both men and women. Sometimes, anger has been so long supressed that we don't feel it on a conscious level. It takes getting into the body, through breath and movement, to release old energies that have caused the qi (energy) to stagnate.

Holding on to anger

Resentment is a complex emotion that mainly consists of low-grade, long-lasting anger and grief that is harboured for days, weeks, years or decades. Like supressed anger, resentment lives as an emotional charge kept inside the body, a permanent fixture of your psyche, impacting your beliefs, relationships and how you interact in the world.

You might believe that if you stay resentful, the person you are resentful towards will experience the same hurt as they inflicted and might understand what it was like for you or the victim you are advocating for. Unfortunately, the energy behind the resentment you hold will never reach your 'enemy', but rather is kept inside you, squeezing like a boa constrictor around your energy body.

From the Chinese medicine perspective, it is essential that qi moves freely, like the way a breeze blows from an open door through a window. Resentment is like closing the windows and doors of your heart. In the process of shutting down energetically, even if only to one person, you lock off some part of you that has the capacity for love and understanding. Also, causing qi to stagnate can lead to various forms of chronic illness. Resentment, in the end, is like drinking your own poison.

The forgiveness process can take time, and usually involves processing the grief behind the past event and summoning a deep well of compassion for yourself and the perpetrator of the original hurt.

Substance use and depression

One of the common strategies for suppressing the feelings that the liver wants to move for you is through the use of substances. Alcohol and, if legally available, marijuana are two very common substances that work temporarily to ease emotional pain but can cause long-term problems for the liver. Alcohol impacts the liver on a physical level, while cannabis impacts the liver on a spiritual level, clouding over the Hun's aspirations with apathy and inhibition.

The reason so many of us turn to substances is to suppress feelings that are uncomfortable or overwhelming. Many of us have not been taught how to feel feelings or regulate them, so substances seem the best option.

The issue with suppressing emotions is that it ultimately leads to various physical and energetic imbalances. Because the liver is responsible for regulating emotions, suppressing any feeling – be it anger, grief, sorrow or disappointment – can result in stagnation of qi and blood flow. When our qi and blood become stagnant, qi is not free to flow around the body to provide nourishment, which increases heat and leads to inflammation. In addition to the physical consequences of the body's inflammatory response, suppressing negative emotions also means suppressing positive emotions like joy, gratitude and love. It is impossible to selectively feel only the good emotions; when we choose not to experience anger or grief, we unknowingly choose to numb ourselves to all emotions. The consequence of long-term emotional suppression is depression. As the liver's energy is suppressed, its spirit, the Hun, no longer provides us with dreams and visions for a brighter future, causing us to lose hope. This can create a negative feedback loop that can keep you stuck in a fairly dark place.

It is important to remember, as you read this book, that suppressing feelings, holding resentments, using substances, bursting into a rage, are all unconscious energy patterns that have built up over time as a part of your unique survival strategy. It is not your fault, and you do not need to get stuck in a cycle of self-blame. Instead, celebrate when you recognize an energy pattern in you that is asking to be worked with. If you found that this chapter describes some of the ways you get stuck, perhaps pick one exercise from the Soul Work section and stick with it, perhaps working alongside a therapist, teacher or mentor. It is important not to read this book and slip into a self-improvement project, however, but simply to bring the connection of the liver energy to what you notice about yourself. Ask yourself: How do I want to love my liver more? In what ways can I nourish the Hun soul and my imaginative capacities? How can I embrace feeling the wide array of emotions without being taken over by them? How can I hold myself and others with more compassion and love?

Flavours of anger

As I stated above, anger is a protection mechanism, and this can take on different flavours depending on the circumstances of our life.

Jealousy and envy are difficult expressions of anger that, at the core, are very vulnerable because they are usually rooted in a fear (related to the kidneys) of not being enough or having enough. Jealousy, specifically, is anger mixed with fear and worry about losing the person you love to someone else, while envy is anger and fear surrounding not having something that someone else possesses.

Guilt and shame are expressions of anger turned inward towards yourself. If you partake in behaviour that causes harm, the Hun will detect it, and the natural feelings that result are remorse, regret or guilt. These emotions signal that you have crossed your own moral boundary. Guilt is not inherently bad, because it can correct behaviour that is not in alignment with your highest values. A little bit of guilt is good – it is the Hun's way of helping us to course-correct.

Shame is different. Shame turns your 'wrong' behaviour to inherent 'wrongness'. Instead of a firm parental voice of skilful self-leadership, shame happens when your inner critic goes on a rampage – overemphasizing your mistakes and denying your worth with aggressive self-denigration. While guilt says, 'I will try better next time, and I am sorry', shame says, 'I am a bad person, why did I even try?'. The energy of shame causes us to collapse back into ourselves and hide who we are, which immobilizes growth and creativity.

The liver energy and Hun spirit want you to grow into your most full and authentic self-expression. Shame suppresses growth, which will lead to qi stagnation in the liver, and more anger/shame energy spinning you into a negative loop. With shame, it helps to really talk about it with a friend or therapist. Shame is stronger when it stays secret, and can be defused faster with a loving and non-judgmental witness.

Imagination tension

Working with the imagination and the growing force of the liver energy is a balancing act between moving forward with your vision, while at the same time not being consumed by your goals. The human imagination creates a constant tension between what is and what could be, and being in this tension can be challenging: it can create impatience and frustration when you are too attached to 'what could be' and can create apathy when you are lagging back into 'what is'.

When the hope of 'what could be' takes us over, aggression and frustration can arise. In being so focused on your goal, it is impossible to see anything else other than the outcome you want to create. Everything and anything that gets in the way of your goal becomes an annoyance. You become short with the ones you love, and impatient. This way of being is overly yang, and it can suck the joy out of your journey.

On the other hand, if you are always lagging back in the 'what is', then you will be missing the vision of where you are going, and can get marooned in old patterns and habits that aren't of service to your Tao. This creates stagnation and a life without any clear direction. This, again, can lead to depression and, quite literally, a life without colour. Some people think that spiritual practice is always about being in the present. A lot of the time it is, but the wood phase and the liver spirit teach us that stepping into the coloured world of our imagination is the only place, personally and collectively, where we can dream a new world into being.

Another place you can get stuck is in the fantasy world itself. You might have a highly developed imagination with tons of ideas, but you struggle to act on any of them. The inability to make decisions can also keep you spinning in the imagination, which can indicate a deficiency in the gallbladder energy. If you have trouble grounding ideas, this can be a good indication that the Hun is overly active, and other organ energies, such as the stomach and lungs, could need some attention.

What I have found helpful to balance the Hun and imagination in my own system, is to fully accept the tension of the imagination. To understand that being present does not mean we do not have ambition, and that having ambition does not mean we need to be stressed out about the outcome.

Remember that when we arrive at our destination, there will always be that tension because new possibilities are infinite. Just like the cedar tree that grows until the day she dies, we reach our branches up to the heavens until our final breath. Knowing that the tension of idealism is the nature of being human might help you settle into the present moment as you grow, and, without urgency or rush, you imagine, hope, dream and courageously step forward without too much concern about the outcome.

Following our Tao is about dancing in the space between what is and what could be, with hope as the music and the steady beat of our heart as the drum.

Symptoms

Take a look at the symptoms opposite, which can arise when the liver and gallbladder are thrown off. If you notice any of these as themes in your life, especially if you experience one symptom in each category, it might indicate your liver and gallbladder need some love!

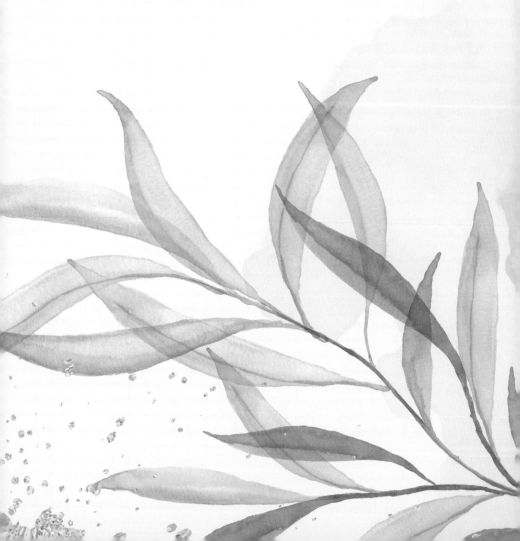

PHYSICAL

❋ headaches/migraines especially in the temples and behind the eyes

❋ painful menstruation

❋ gynaecological conditions (endometriosis, fibroids, polycystic ovary syndrome)

❋ tight neck and shoulders

❋ dry or red eyes, poor vision, floaters in vision

❋ tendonitis

❋ waking during the night between 1 a.m. and 3 a.m.

❋ nail fungus, brittle or ridged nails

ENERGETIC

❋ irritability, anger

❋ feeling impatient and rushed

❋ feeling overly competitive

❋ sporadic outbursts of emotions and mood swings

❋ being self-critical

❋ having a 'shout' sound to the voice, or a voice that carries a long distance

❋ craving alcohol

❋ bouts of depression and hopelessness

SPIRITUAL

❋ inability to envision the future

❋ being directionless or apathetic about the future

❋ struggling to make decisions or to 'pull the trigger' on decisions you make

❋ being overly focused on the future and outcome of goals

❋ lack imagination and dreams, day and night

❋ feeling as though your life is stagnant

SOUL WORK
FROM ANGER TO ALTRUISM

The soul work for the liver is an invitation to allow your emotions to be felt and moved. The invitation is for you to redirect the energy of anger, frustration or resentment into creativity, compassion and a vision for a new future, both for yourself and the collective.

Physical Soul Work

At a physical level, the liver is greatly affected by our diet and level of physical activity. As the liver plays a crucial role in the smooth flow of qi, if we do not engage in regular physical movement, the qi becomes stagnant, leading to stress on the liver. So, it is important to incorporate daily physical activity into your routine to ensure the proper movement of liver qi. Engaging in more vigorous exercises, such as running, cycling or strength training, on occasion can also be beneficial.

Additionally, it is crucial to consume foods that support the liver, such as fresh green leafy vegetables, including kale, collards, bok choy, Chinese cabbage (napa greens), leek, daikon tops, green radish tops, turnip tops, dandelion greens and lettuces. These foods have an upward-moving energy that the liver particularly appreciates. Although this book doesn't focus on nutrition, it's important to mention that diet greatly affects the psychological expression of this energy. Consulting a Chinese medicine practitioner or nutrition expert can be helpful in determining which foods will specifically support your body and constitution.

One of the most direct ways we can help our liver on a physical, energetic and spiritual level without seeking counsel from a nutrition expert is through reducing our exposure to toxins and mind-altering substances, such as alcohol, recreational drugs, pharmaceutical drugs and cannabis.

EXERCISE
LIVER MERIDIAN STRETCHING
AND VISUALIZATION PRACTICE

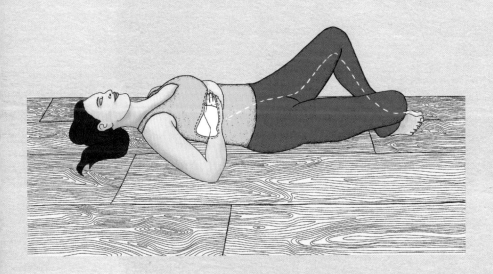

This practice stretches the fascia tissue along the liver energy channels and, when combined with your intention, can be a powerful way to break up energy stagnation through the liver organ energy system. This practice also encourages deep relaxation, which helps encourage the flow of qi through the body. This can be a quiet and nurturing practice you can do before bed or upon waking. For further reading on postures that stretch meridians, please see the additional resources section on 'yin yoga' at the back of this book.

1 Begin by finding a comfortable place to lie down, either in your bed or on the floor on a mat or carpet. If it helps you to relax, you can play soft music, or light an incense or candle. Bend your knees and bring the soles of your feet together with your knees apart. Adjust your body until you feel a mild to medium stretch along the inside line of your legs and into your groin. You want to feel a mild stretch while also relaxing completely. If the stretch is too intense, place pillows, cushions or yoga blocks under your thighs.

2 Place both of your hands over your liver, which is under your ribcage on your right side. Trace your attention along the liver meridian, which runs from the inside of your big toe, up the inner ankle, up the inner leg and across the groin, and finally into the body towards the liver.

3 Start by taking long, slow, deep breaths. You might imagine that you were relaxing somewhere in nature where you feel safe and supported: maybe in a forest, in the mountains or in a tropical location. As you inhale, imagine breathing in a mystical green mist that carries fresh energy to nourish the liver. You might imagine this green energy carrying virtuous qualities, such as imagination, compassion, creativity and patience. Visualize this energy flowing like a river from your big toes along the liver meridians and towards your liver. As you exhale, breath out of your mouth, releasing any toxic energy from your liver. You can imagine a black cloud exiting your mouth as you release any feelings of anger, frustration, resentment, jealousy and physical disease. Inhale fresh, brilliant green qi from your feet to your liver, and exhale out of your mouth, releasing. Each breath is energetically 'cleaning' your liver. Repeat for a minimum of nine breaths, or a maximum of five minutes.

4 Draw your knees back together, perhaps hugging your knees into your chest or rocking your legs from right to left to release any tension that has built up. Extend your legs straight down and notice how you feel.

Energetic Soul Work

Working with the liver on an energetic level is about transmuting the upward explosive energy of anger and all of its flavours: rage, frustration, resentment, shame, blame and self-criticism. We work with this energy through first acknowledging it as a 'felt sense' in the body, then relating to it with curiosity and care, and then giving that energy somewhere to go that is not harmful for yourself or another. Remember: the energy of anger has to go somewhere, otherwise it will stagnate in the body and lead to some form of imbalance. On the other hand, overindulging in anger promotes the habit of turning away from yourself and always blaming the outside world for your unhappiness. When you do this, you avoid taking responsibility for your own feelings.

If you are someone who never experiences anger, it might be helpful to wonder about your relationship to the wood energy in general. Is there ever a time you wish you would have spoken up or defended someone or something?

For the gallbladder, the soul work requires nurturing the energy required to make decisions and not waver with them. Decisions require taking a stand for something. If you notice you are overly hesitant, you might practise making small decisions, such as what to cook for dinner or which jeans to wear. Practise making these small decisions without looking back. Notice how that energy feels compared to wavering back and forth or staying in the place of not deciding anything.

EXERCISE
CALLING ON THE DRAGON

I work with anger using the acronym DRAGON. In Chinese culture, the dragon is believed to have an innate ability to see beyond the present and into the future. It is often regarded as a symbol of wisdom and foresight. When we call upon the dragon, we are calling upon our capacity to hold ourselves compassionately, until we can see again with our wisdom eyes. At the same time, we call upon the dragon to allow the anger to move through us and honour what its energy needs, without hurting ourselves or others.

1 Drop In
The first step to working with anger, especially if it is expressed towards someone else, is to notice that you are feeling it and drop into your body so you can get to know its energy. Anger is an energy that will continue to poison you unless you disarm it, and in order to do this, you have to turn the attention from outside to inside. It helps in this first step to drop the gaze and/or close the eyes.

2 Recognize
The second step is to recognize what kind of anger is present. Can you name it as rage, resentment, jealousy? Is the anger directed at yourself or another person? If you struggle to feel anger, maybe you are still slightly annoyed or impatient, or perhaps there is another feeling hidden underneath.

3 Analyze

Take a few deep breaths and notice where anger shows up in your body. Is there a shape, colour, texture or flavour to the energy? Do you feel anger in your fists, your belly, chest or head?

4 Greet

Can you greet your anger with curiosity and understanding? As a strong energetic messenger, what does it want you to know? What is it protecting? Is there a part of you that is hurt which is being the energy of anger? What is the unmet need that the anger is trying to communicate to you?

5 Oxygen

Take a minimum of three deep breaths into the feeling of hurt/disappointment/fear or whatever emotion is behind your anger. I recommend placing a hand somewhere on your body and having compassion for the part of you the anger has been protecting.

6 New Direction

Where does that energy want to go? Perhaps you need to go for a run or start a creative project. Can you use that energy to push into a new direction, into a new vision for your future or the future of the collective, or, simply, a new way of being or seeing the situation?

Spiritual Soul Work

On a spiritual level, the soul work for the liver revolves around supporting, training and enhancing the imagination, while allowing the critical and sceptical aspects of your mind that say, 'That isn't realistic!', to take a step back. Forms of meditation that offer guided imagery are helpful for this, as well as enquiring into night-time dream messages, daydream messages and visions.

On the spirit level, the liver is about training you to see possibilities that might seem radically optimistic. It is about exercising your inner vision and creative capacity, and satisfying the human need for beauty. Going to an art museum or participating in creative endeavours, such as painting or sculpture, will help nourish the soul. Like the palm reader in the line-up of war prisoners, who dreamed the impossible into being (see page 80), so, too, do we have the capacity to dream and conjure up ideas that may or may not come to fruition. From these ideas, possibilities start to unfold and the energy of renewal is activated.

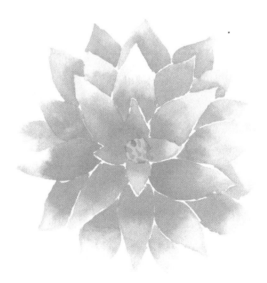

EXERCISE
JOURNALLING

This journalling activity is meant to exercise your imagination. If you are not a visual person, this can take a bit of practice. You can also invite other senses in, such as smells, sounds or a felt sense in your body. If writing isn't your thing, try drawing or recording a voice note, or talking about it with a friend.

1 Take a few moments to close your eyes with your journal by your side. You can sit comfortably or lie down and contemplate the following questions:

> What would my life look like if I were living in alignment with my Tao?
>
> What would it feel like, who would be around me, where would I live?
>
> What job would I have?
>
> Who would my friends be?
>
> How would I spend my time?

Notice which images feel the 'truest' in your heart (see the Heart Reading exercise on pages 67–8). Take a moment to write or draw your responses.

2 Now lean back and contemplate the following questions:

> What qualities will I need to cultivate in order for this to come to fruition?
>
> What qualities or habits will I have to let go of?
>
> What kind of support will I need along the way?

Write or draw your responses.

3 Ask yourself:

> What is one small decision I can make that brings me closer to living in the direction of my vision?

CHAPTER 3
Ground of Intention

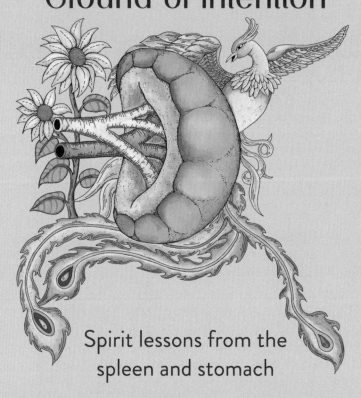

Spirit lessons from the
spleen and stomach

'If your mind becomes firm like a rock and no
longer shakes, in a world where everything is
shaking, your mind will be your greatest friend...'

Therigatha (*Verses of the Elder Nuns*, c. 600–300 BCE)

I wake abruptly in the middle of the night, startled by the sensation of the ground trembling beneath me. The bed frame wobbles back and forth, swaying in sync with the earth's movements. The artwork on the wall becomes loose, inching closer to the ground, as the windows rattle, echoing like thunder throughout my bamboo *casa*. The earth's power shakes me to my bones, destabilizing my core. In a state of panic, I quickly sit up. I have never been in an earthquake before. I am on the coastline of Lake Atitlan in Guatemala, practicing qigong and meditation at a hermitage. I have been in solitude for several weeks, so I pinch myself to be sure this is not a hallucination. When I realize that I am indeed experiencing an earthquake, and one of significant magnitude, my initial instinct is to run down the stairs and outside, and put my feet on the earth. Perhaps I could lie down on the ground where there will be less movement? Then I remember that it is the ground itself that is trembling, and that I cannot seek refuge in it. I come to the realization that stability, in this moment, does not exist. I stay in my bed, palms gripping the sheets, enduring the wave of the earth's quake and the aftershocks that rumbled until dawn.

The earthquake taught me many things that night, but perhaps the most poignant lesson was it highlighted the silent way the earth element supports every facet of our life. The earth is what we stand on, the foundation on which we build our homes, the source of our sustenance and the stage on which our life unfolds. Like the earth element, its associated organs – the stomach and spleen – offer us stability, nurturance and constancy. When balanced, the spleen and stomach energy doesn't move anywhere, but rather transforms and supports where we are standing. The movement of the stomach and spleen is one of grounded transformation: receiving nutrients from food and, quite literally, building the body through the assimilation of food to flesh.

According to Chinese medicine, the spleen is responsible for qualities that are foundational for human functioning: our thoughts, intellect and the formation of our intentions. When our spleen is compromised, we may experience feelings of worry, excessive thinking and a lack of centredness, balance and comfort in our own bodies. The earth element, which rules the central direction, serves as a centring force, keeping us focused on our intentions. It provides the stability needed to transform our goals, inspired by our inner wisdom (Shen) and ideas (Hun), into something practical and tangible in our everyday lives. The earth element also acts as a maypole that tethers us to our centre, and when things get rocky, we can return to it, finding stability even 'in a world, where everything is shaking'.

ASSOCIATIONS

Spirit: Yi

Element: Earth

Yin organ: Spleen

Yang organ: Stomach

Animal: Phoenix

Season: Late summer

Colour: Gold

Direction: Centre

Voice tone: Sing

Negative emotion: Worry, excess sympathy

Balanced emotion: Trust, contentment

Physical function: Digestion, the production of blood and qi

Energetic function: Self-care, assimilation and digestion of information and experiences, clear thought process

Spirit function: Intention setting, devotion, constancy

PHYSICAL FUNCTION
THE PRODUCTION OF BLOOD AND QI

On a physical level, the spleen is an organ about the size of your fist and it is located on the upper left side of your abdomen. It is positioned next to your stomach and behind your left ribs. From the Western medical perspective, the spleen is part of your lymphatic system and aids your immune system. You can technically live without a spleen, and many people do, because the liver will take over the functions that are vital for survival.

The spleen plays a more significant role in Chinese medicine, as it is responsible for assimilating nutrients into the energy the body needs. From the Chinese medicine perspective, even if your spleen is removed, you still have spleen energy. It is important to note that the spleen and the pancreas are considered the same organ in Chinese medicine, and are the yin organs to the yang organ of the stomach. Together, these organs govern all digestive processes that transform raw food into blood and energy for our limbs and large muscles. When the spleen is compromised, the qi (energy) weakens, which can result in lethargy. Symptoms of a weakened spleen may include a poor appetite, sluggish digestion, indigestion and loose, watery stools. While the liver is responsible for moving blood, the spleen is responsible for producing it. When the spleen's qi is weak, a person may easily bruise or experience problems with bleeding.

The stomach is a large hollow 'J'-shaped organ and lives under your ribcage on the left side. It is responsible for receiving food and secreting enzymes to break up the food before it is passed into the small intestine. In Chinese medicine, it is crucial for the stomach's physical function that energy moves downwards, allowing food to be absorbed and transformed into energy itself. A typical imbalance in the stomach occurs when the energy becomes 'rebellious' and moves in the opposite direction. Rebellious qi in the stomach shows up as nausea, vomiting, excessive burping and indigestion. In extreme cases, being unable to swallow is also a sign of rebellious stomach energy.

In general, any problems with digestion will somehow be related to the earth element and stomach and spleen function in Chinese medicine.

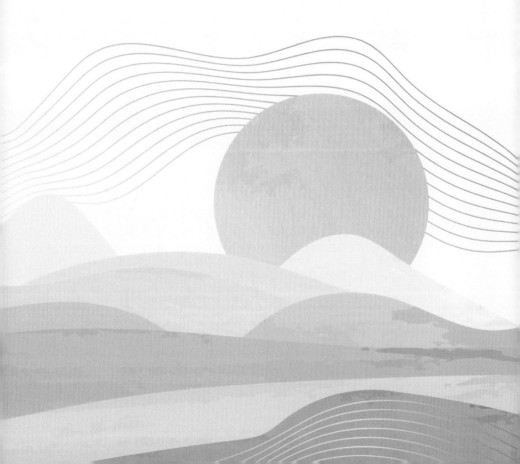

ENERGETIC FUNCTION
PSYCHOLOGICAL DIGESTION AND NOURISHMENT

The energy of the earth phase, along with the stomach and spleen energy, forms a spiralling motion around our centre. The earth energy represents the centre direction on the compass, and unlike the heart that moves out and the liver that moves up, the spleen moves away from our centre but actually strengthens the qi around it. Just as the earth spirals round its axis, this energy helps to harmonize the forces of yin and yang and facilitate their transformation. The spleen's steadfast magnetism plays a role in grounding us in the material plane.

When this spiralling energy becomes disorganized, it creates knots that can lead to feelings of worry and pensiveness. However, when this energy is balanced, it fosters the emotions of trust and contentment. It provides a sense of being centred and nourished in life, allowing for stability and harmony.

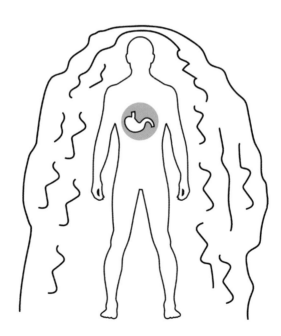

If the physical role of the spleen and stomach is about transforming nutrients from food into nourishment, its energetic role is to receive, break down and transform psychological and emotional material into nourishment for the mind. While we think of nutrients only as food, there are other forms of nutrients that we take in through all our five senses. We are consuming mental and emotional stimuli all the time: the media on your phone or TV, the music you listen to, the conversations you have with your friends and co-workers, the books that you read, the billboard you drive by each day. Anything that comes into your field of consciousness is consumed and integrated into your memory and knowledge base – and it literally has to be 'digested'.

Zen master, Thich Nhat Hanh, calls these 'nutriments' in his book *Silence*, and notes that just like watching what we eat so that our body stays healthy, so too do we need to watch what we consume through these other senses to maintain a healthy mind. We can feel nourished by an inspiring book, a hug from a friend, a compliment, a beautiful walk in the garden. Taking these things in and allowing ourselves to be nourished is the role of these organs. Other 'nutriments', just like food, can make us feel 'sick', such as overindulging in the news, scrolling on social media and comparing yourself to others, or participating in a gossipy conversation at work. Working with the stomach and spleen energies is a lot about paying attention to what you consume.

The stomach and the spleen have slightly different roles in digesting experience. The stomach receives the nutrients, while the spleen transforms them. The ability to 'take in' information when learning something new, for example, is the energetic function of the stomach, while being able to assimilate and apply that new knowledge into a thought and a task would be the role of the spleen. Both are required for the digestion process.

Thinking

One of the things that the spleen transforms experience into is thoughts. In Chinese medicine, all thoughts are a product of the spleen. Just as the spleen transforms food into blood, it also generates the thoughts that shape not only our identity but also our values and belief systems. Once 'nutriments' are absorbed, they are presented and known to the heart, and the Shen can reflect back what that input means to the innermost core of our being. Once 'digested', the spleen produces feedback through mental activity. In essence, a large part of our psyche is formed through our thinking, as famously stated by Descartes: 'I think, therefore I am.' Although our thoughts do not define who we are on an ultimate level, they serve as a bridge between our consciousness (spirit/Tao) and the physical world (body/material realm). It is through the medium of thought that our intellect takes root, intentions are formed and our Tao can manifest from a mere dream into something tangible in the material world.

I have to stress that thinking is a function largely conditioned by what you consume – and while thinking can be skilful when guided by the heart, it does not always reflect your deepest values or meaning, especially when the thoughts are automatic. We have thousands of thoughts throughout the day, and a lot of them are just thought without much substance or relevance to our Tao. For example, if you spend the weekend binge-watching your favourite TV show, chances are you will find yourself thinking about the characters, maybe unconsciously having the theme song stuck in your head, or perhaps even dreaming about it.

Home and routines

So, the stomach and spleen offer stability and are nourished by stability. Having a steady home and putting down roots somewhere can help to nourish the stomach and spleen energy. Travelling or moving constantly, or flying a lot for work, can have a destabilizing effect on the earth element and the stomach and spleen energies. I know personally that my digestion is off when I travel, and has been bothersome when I have been in states of uncertainty about my home. Something as simple as unpacking after a long trip can help settle and root the stomach and spleen energy. Getting back into a consistent routine, not only with meals but with daily activities, will help nourish this organ.

On an energetic level, these organs also relate to the home and being rooted somewhere. The stomach and spleen are nourished by all matters domestic, such as setting up a house and being settled in a place for some time. They are nourished by a warm home, with lots of food in the fridge, warm blankets and even an inviting 'welcome' sign on the door.

Caretaking and generosity

Since the spleen and stomach are ruled by the earth element, it is unsurprising that they relate intimately with the mother archetype. The 'mother' nourishes and shows up unconditionally with anything and everything that we need: food, shelter, care or love. Similarly, one of the functions of the spleen/stomach is to take care of others and yourself – you do not need to physically be a mother to embody the mother archetype. The caring that is related to the stomach and spleen is not just a warm fuzzy feeling of love, but one that physically shows up and does something. This is the love that wipes the puke off the floor when your dog is sick, or drives ageing parents to their medical appointment. Caretaking is, like the mother archetype, selfless and without an agenda; it is generous and consistent, and is guided by the needs of the person or people you are serving.

The emotion that is often associated with the spleen is sympathy, and this can express through the act of caretaking. However, as we will go over in the Soul Work section, it is equally as important to take care of yourself, because it is impossible to serve when you are undernourished. Being overly sympathetic and 'taking on the world's problems' can be a common imbalance in the spleen energy. When this energy is balanced, there is an equal ability to give support and receive it.

SPIRITUAL FUNCTION
INTENTION

The spirit of the spleen and stomach is known as the Yi. This is often translated as 'intellect', and it is where human volition is born. The Yi is where your Tao starts to formulate into a clear and solid intention and shows up in your daily actions. The Yi is an important spirit because it lives at the centre, between your divine instincts (Shen and Hun) and your body's instincts (Po and Zhi). It is realistic, practical, humble and devoted.

The spirit animal associated with the spleen is the phoenix, which is not an ordinary bird. It has the characteristics of a chicken, swan, snake and fish, with wings made of ivory horns and the ability to consume various types of bamboo and wine, assimilating them into energy for its flight. The phoenix is adorned with feathers in the five elemental colours: blue/black, red, gold, green and white, and has the essential human virtues written all over its body: righteousness on its back, faithfulness on its belly and love across its chest. The yin and yang nature of the phoenix represents the Yi's capacity to fly between the yin impulses of the body and the yang illumination of the spirit, and to choose actions that align with your soul's true path. Its multicoloured feathers symbolize the culmination of all the organ energies and the gifts they bring through our focused presence and unwavering intentions.

The phoenix also teaches us the importance of balancing what is right for our soul's path with virtue. It reminds us that a true intention is not genuine if it does not lead with loving kindness. In the Buddhist tradition, which is inseparable from the evolution of Chinese medicine, 'right intention' or 'right thought' is a pillar of the spiritual path. It is taught that if we lead with intentions fuelled by lust, ill will and hostility, it will ultimately lead to suffering for ourselves and others. On the other hand, if we lead with the intention of renunciation (letting go), goodwill and compassion, it will lead to greater freedom for ourselves and others. The phoenix serves as a powerful reminder for us to continually re-evaluate our intentions, particularly those we deem as 'good'. It prompts us to reflect on whether these intentions are truly grounded in virtue, or if they are driven by ego or other self-serving motives.

Truth vow

It is important to differentiate between an intention and a goal. Goals represent the liver's long-term vision – a goal implies some sort of destination and stretches us into new possibility. Intention, on the other hand, is more constant. It is anchored to the Shen's truth and acts based on that truth, regardless of the circumstances it is faced with. The Vedic word for intention is *sankalpa*, which literally translates as 'truth vow'. I find this translation fitting when it comes to understanding the essence of the spleen: the heart holds the truth, while the Yi is dedicated to that truth no matter what happens. While the goal is the vision of where we aim to be, intention drives each step we take towards that destination and also serves as the underlying motivation for why we pursue it.

One way we can differentiate between a goal and an intention is to remember that intention is the force that moves energy. There is a saying in qigong, that 'qi follows Yi' or 'energy flows where our intention goes'. When we intend something, the energy flows there. Let's do a little experiment for a moment. Think about bending your left elbow. Don't actually move the elbow but think about bending it. Notice how the energy starts to collect around the elbow. This is the way energy works: it is moved by the mind. On a larger scale, if we intend in a devoted way to what we want to create from our heart, the energy of our life will start to flow towards what we care most about and, over time, we start to create that reality.

Let's say you go on a hike with a friend. Your goal is to reach the top and enjoy the views. However, your intention goes beyond that – it's about connecting and having a great time. Throughout the journey, your intention remains constant. You engage in conversations, capture pictures and take breaks when needed, always ensuring a good time. While the goal of reaching the top propels you forwards, the deeper intention of putting energy into your friendship remains unchanged, regardless of the outcome. This illustrates the difference between Hun and Yi – Hun pushes us towards what we believe is possible, while Yi takes steady steps, keeping us focused on the heart's truth. Even if things don't go as planned, Yi helps us stay steady and committed, never losing our centre.

So, we can ask our heart: what matters? And then we can ask the liver: what would that look like? But to bring what matters to the heart into matter takes a tremendous amount of energy and a deep dive into mundane, nitty gritty detail. It is like planting a garden – you have to plant the seeds and tend to it day in, day out. If you only water it once, the garden will die. This is the same for anything we want to create in life, whether that is a project, a habit or an internal quality. Doing something once will not create change. This is simply how energy works. To bring something from high frequency (insight and thought) into low frequency (physical existence) the energy pattern must repeat itself until it crystallizes into form.

This is true for any quality you want to create in yourself. If you want to be less of an anxious person, you cannot just practise deep breathing or meditation once: the power is in repetition. Once is never enough. There is nothing more powerful than small steady steps tethered to your heart's deepest truths.

Trust

Trust, both in oneself and others, is energetically connected to the stomach and spleen. We have no choice but to trust the earth, which is mostly stable beneath our feet. On a spiritual level, when we align our intentions with virtue and keep the Tao in mind, we become more trustworthy to ourselves and others. A lot of my therapy clients will often tell me, 'I don't feel grounded' or 'I don't know how to ground myself'. It is important to remember that groundedness isn't just about physical stability, but rather internal stability. This internal ground is formed by our unwavering intention, acting as a guiding principle for our lives. Even in times of turmoil, like my experience in an earthquake, we can always return to our energetic centre, which resides within our own volition. The truer our intentions are, the more we can trust ourselves and maintain our centredness, even when life lacks stability.

Doing something once will not create change.
This is simply how energy works.

To bring something from high frequency
(insight and thought) into low frequency
(physical existence) the energy pattern
must repeat itself until it crystalizes into form.

It is your habits, the little things you do
each day, that will transform your life.

WHERE YOU GET STUCK
RUMINATION AND WORRY

The negative emotion that is associated with the earth element and the stomach and spleen is worry. On an energetic level, worry happens when a lot of thinking is produced but doesn't lead to any action – instead, the Yi moves round and round in circles. Because 'qi follows Yi', the qi then literally 'knots', creating blockage in and around the stomach and spleen area. Worry can be a result of excess sympathy, as in the case of a worried mother who says, 'I was worried sick'. The sick feeling in your stomach when you are worried or ruminating about something is the result of this energy knotting.

Rumination is slightly different to worry because it can sustain any difficult emotion, such as jealousy, anger, rage or fear. Emotions only last as a psychosomatic experience for about 90 seconds – it is re-thinking about the thing that upset you, without doing anything about it, that causes the emotion to become chronic. In the liver chapter, we talked about the importance of emotions moving in order to prevent stagnation. And while we want to feel our emotions, ruminating keeps us stuck in them, rather than promoting movement.

What I have found in my own experience with earth energy imbalances and rumination and worry is that there is a lack of trust beneath the worry – either not trusting your own intentions or an inability to trust others. Playing out possible 'what if' scenarios over and over can give the illusion you have control over the situation, when, in reality, it is just making you sick.

Inability to receive

The earth element and stomach/spleen energy relate to the season of late summer. It represents the time of harvest, abundance, nourishment and celebration. One of the most common imbalances of stomach energy you might notice within yourself is the inability to receive. On a physical level, this shows up as nausea, vomiting, burping and indigestion, but on an emotional level, this looks like not being able to receive the nourishment of life's bounty.

Let's take a look at a few examples of how this might show up in life. Imagine that you treat yourself to a spa day for self-care. However, when you arrive at the spa, you end up bringing your phone with you to the relaxation lounge and become consumed with thoughts about all the things you need to do, instead of enjoying the experience of your facial or the spa music. Even though you are physically at the spa, you might only let a fraction of the experience nourish your mind and body. Clearing the mind of clutter so that we can allow our body to be nourished by experiences of self-care can help with the receiving process.

Another example of not fully receiving is failing to celebrate the completion of a task. Each time we complete something offers an opportunity to nourish our mind. Whether it is as big as a graduation or as small as going to the grocery store, taking time to revel in that completion can help us feel more nourished on a daily basis. Moving on to the next thing without that breath of appreciation can make life feel like an endless treadmill of 'to-do' lists, without any time to savour the fruit of our intentions.

Another commonplace way the inability to receive shows up is in relationships. In my own experience, I noticed a curious pattern between my partner and I. Whenever he would express his love for me, I would automatically respond with 'love you too' before he had even finished speaking. I realized that by immediately reciprocating this way, I was deflecting his love instead of truly embracing it. Now, I make a conscious effort to pause and fully absorb his love without feeling the need to immediately reciprocate. Similarly, when someone compliments me, I make a conscious effort to truly take it in, and even allow myself to feel the discomfort of receiving appreciation, before saying 'Thank you' or responding with another compliment.

Our inability to receive can leave us feeling undernourished by life. Are you able to receive love from family and friends, or accept support when you need it? Do you struggle to accept compliments, gifts or appreciation? Even if you are able to receive a compliment, do you take the time to let it sink in and nourish you?

Too much

Another way earth element imbalance shows up is a general milieu of overindulgence. This can show up in any form of consumption: eating, watching TV, shopping, talking, thinking. You might even start to notice your house being full of clutter. As I mentioned before, overindulgence can be a result of not fully letting in the bounty of life's inherent richness, leaving us hungry. It can also be an unconscious coping mechanism to numb painful emotions from the past. We cannot selectively feel our emotions. When we block painful ones, we also block beautiful ones. Blocking beautiful feelings keeps us undernourished by experiences and relationships, leaving us hungry, and so we take refuge in the temporary fullness that eating, shopping or binge-watching Netflix provides.

No harvest

On a spiritual level, the most common imbalance with the stomach energy is the inability for thought to follow through into an action: you don't do what you say you are going to do. I notice this happening frequently in the spiritual community among yogis and individuals who are deeply committed to developing their spirit. While they may have a strong connection to their Tao, there is often a lack of practicality or ability to manifest their spiritual ideals into reality. They generate numerous ideas and dream big aspirations, but struggle to focus or commit to one thing, resulting in ideas remaining as mere ideas and dreams as mere dreams. Consequently, they live their lives in the clouds, instead of grounding their spirituality in their everyday existence. And because they are stuck in the idea phase of a project or inner quality they want to cultivate, nothing ever comes to fruition. As a result, they are also left undernourished by life, because there is never actually a harvest on the earthly plane.

Additionally, when we remain immersed in the realm of higher spirits (Shen and Hun), it is impossible to ground our intentions. This results in a lack of focus and stability, causing us to easily be swayed by the vicissitudes of life. For those addicted to meditation and spiritual life, there can be the tendency to seek refuge in ethereal realms, where things seem easier. However, staying in the spirit dimensions prevents us from fully engaging in the human experience, which is what our soul chose as a vehicle for growth. The Taoists suggest that spiritual life is not about the ascent into another reality, but the decent of our Shen's light to every aspect of our life here on earth. The Yi is the humble spirit that dares to manifest the Shen's truth within the challenging circumstances we find ourselves in. It requires tremendous perseverance, repetition and unwavering dedication to the practical details.

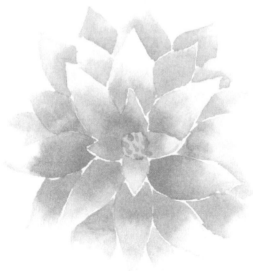

Symptoms

Take a look at the symptoms opposite, which can arise when the spleen and stomach energy are thrown off. If you notice any of these as themes in your life, especially if you experience one symptom in each category, it might indicate your spleen and stomach need some love!

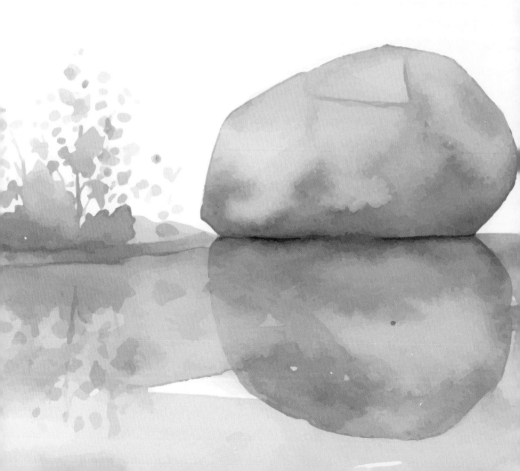

PHYSICAL

* indigestion
* nausea/vomiting
* inability to swallow or keep food down
* fatigue
* brain fog/cannot think clearly
* diarrhea/loose stools
* chronic nose bleeds
* prolapse

ENERGETIC

* overthinking/rumination
* worry
* can't stop talking
* voice has a 'sing-song' intonation
* inability to say no
* putting everyone else's needs before your own
* inability to receive – gifts, compliments, support or love

SPIRITUAL

* disconnected from your centre
* inability to set intentions
* inability to follow through with ideas and plans
* inconsistency in where your energy is going

SOUL WORK
FROM RUMINATION TO RIGHT ACTION

The soul work for the stomach and spleen involves paying attention to what you consume on a physical, energetic and spiritual level, giving yourself appropriate time and space to digest. The spleen invites you to set a strong intention and act from the centre of that intention in all your daily activities.

Physical Soul Work

Like the liver, the spleen and stomach are greatly impacted by the foods we eat. While nutrition is not the emphasis of this book, eating highly processed foods and fast foods that are high in fat and sugar will stress the stomach and spleen.

The spleen energy is stressed not only by what you eat, but how and how much. Remember that the spleen likes stability and routine. Eating irregularly can lead to indigestion, as can eating on the move or while standing up. Part of the soul work of the spleen is to notice your daily habits of stuffing food into your mouth unconsciously, snacking when making supper or even forgetting to eat until you are starving. To nourish your spleen, consider scheduling regular mealtimes where you can sit down and eat mindfully. Remember, qi follows Yi. If your mealtimes are intentional, it is more likely you will be able to digest your food with ease.

Additionally, eating while worried or upset can further throw off our energy. It is said that if we eat when upset, we consume the emotion that is arising, pushing it further into the body. So, can you treat even one meal per day as a sacred and quiet time to be nourished? Lastly, the Taoists say that leaving one-third of the stomach empty helps the movement of qi through this organ so that food can be digested. Do you have to eat until you are stuffed, or can you leave some breathing room?

Another piece of soul work on a physical level that is helpful for the spleen and stomach energy is diaphragmatic breathing. The stomach and spleen energy channels run right through the thoracic diaphragm, which is your main breathing muscle that lives under your ribcage. When we are worried, this is also where the qi likes to knot up, and we tend to tense and restrict around our bellies. I like to think of the diaphragm as the energetic centre, the place where the unconscious and the conscious begin to communicate with each other. Mobilizing the diaphragm helps to mobilize feelings that have been locked away in the body unconsciously so that they can be digested. It can also help to free up the qi that has been knotted through rumination and worry.

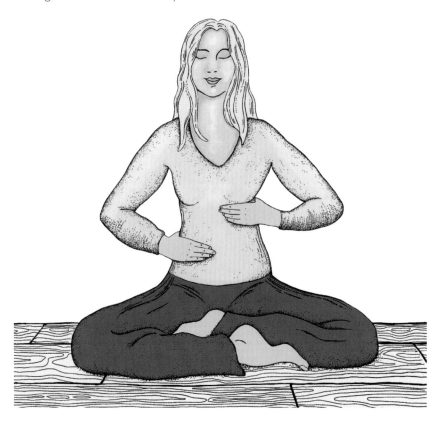

EXERCISE
FINDING YOUR DIAPHRAGM AND ITS CHANNELS

Because the diaphragm sits on top of the organs, each breath acts as a massage, helping up break stagnation and move energy that has been stuck in your organs. It is very common to experience emotions moving as you start to practise this. While this exercise is known as 'belly breathing', we have to remember that mobilizing the diaphragm is more than just the belly lifting up and down. To really move the diaphragm, we want the entire mid-section to stretch and the expansion to be felt in the side and back of the waist too.

1 Start by finding a comfortable place to sit or lie down – whatever works for you. Bring you right hand onto your chest and your left hand onto your abdomen. Notice where your breath is moving most naturally. If your breath is moving under your right hand, and not in your abdomen, chances are you are holding on to a lot of tension in the diaphragm.

2 Next, encourage your breath down into your belly, so that your right hand remains still, and your left hand moves up and down with your breath.

3 Breathe slowly, in through the nose for a count of four or five, and out through the mouth for the same count. Breathing out of the mouth allows for any stagnant energy to leave the body. Repeat for five to nine rounds.

4 Now, slide your hands down to the lower part of each side of your ribcage, where it starts to taper in towards the abdomen. Wrap your hands round this part of your waist, with the thumbs to the back of your body and the four fingers wrapping forward on the sides of the ribs. As you do, inhale, and imagine your diaphragm descending and pushing out into your hands three dimensionally.

5 Take a moment and hold your breath for a few counts, feeling the diaphragm push down on the organs of the abdomen and stretch outward evenly into your hands – front, back and sides. You might even feel a tight or 'stretching' sensation. Exhale slowly out of your mouth. Repeat for three rounds.

6 Next, relax both of your hands down to your abdomen, and breathe in, encouraging this three-dimensional breath, for a slow count of four to five. Breathe out for the same count.

7 This time, breathe in and out of the mouth. Doing this helps to disperse the qi in the lower regions of the body. Repeat for five to nine rounds.

8 Finally, let go of any effort to breathe and return to your natural breathing. Notice how you feel.

Energetic Soul Work

Because thoughts are a product of what we consume, the first piece of energetic-level soul work is to review what you are consuming, and how much. What TV are you watching? Who are you following on social media? Do you overindulge in the news? Consumption also includes visual stimulus in the areas of the home and workplace that you frequently look at. Is there a lot of clutter around you? Cleaning up the clutter in your physical space can help ease feelings of clutter in your inner life as well. Just as the stomach likes to be two-thirds full, giving your mind space to not consume at every moment of every day is vital. Trimming down what you consume on an energetic level will help to declutter the mind and produce thoughts that are attuned with your deeper intentions.

The next piece of soul work for the spleen and stomach on an energetic level is to start to notice what you think. Do your thoughts take you over? Do most of them lead to an action, or do they just spin around in your head? Some thoughts are harmful to consume, such as those that perpetuate jealousy, envy, rage and fear. Thoughts can be addictive and, like food, we consume them, but in the end, they consume us! Spending too much time in the head disconnects us from the body and depletes our energy. Rumination leads to the negative emotion of worry, but is also linked to so many mental health illnesses, including depression and anxiety.

There are a few ways to work with worry and rumination. The first is to do something about what you are worried about. For example, if you are worried about your taxes, is might be a good idea to phone an accountant and start your return papers early. This gives the thought, and the energetic charge behind the thought, somewhere to go. It can also be as simple as phoning the friend who didn't text you back and who you can't stop thinking about.

If there is nothing you can do about the thoughts that are spinning in your head, go deeper beneath the surface level of thinking (the thoughts themselves) and tap into the energy that is driving them. All thoughts require energy to keep going. By focusing on the energy behind our thoughts, we are taking care of ourselves while also freeing ourselves from the endless loop of thoughts that hold us back. Once we connect with this energy, it can be beneficial to find an alternative word or thought that helps us regain stability – such as an affirmation or mantra. The Buddha taught this concept, suggesting that one way to work with thoughts is by replacing them. He uses the metaphor of a carpenter who removes a rotten peg and replaces it with a new one; similarly, we should remove the thoughts that lead us astray and replace them with more constructive ones.

'Whatever you frequently think and ponder upon, that will become the inclination of your mind.'

The Buddha

EXERCISE
CHANGING THE PEG

This practice is for when you find yourself ruminating or in a state of worry. Jealousy and anger can also be sustained by rumination, so this practice can help if you find yourself swirling in any such negative emotion.

1 Stop where you are and bring your attention to your head. Close your eyes and listen to what your thoughts are saying. What does the voice in your head sound like? Is it harsh, whiny or childish-sounding? Take a moment to get to know the thought without being the thought.

2 Next, drop your attention from your head to your torso, between the neck and the sitting bones. What do you feel in your body as your mind produces these thoughts? Drop from the content of the thought and sink down into the body's 'felt sense' of it. Get specific on the location, the shape, the colour and texture.

3 Then use the deep breathing method on page 120 to let this energy move. Continue to stay connected to the body and avoid falling back into the story and thought loop of the emotion. Instead, stay with the body sensation. Now ask that sensation what it needs? Is there a gesture, action or piece of self-care that you can follow through on?

4 Lastly, choose a word or phrase to replace the ruminating thought and soothe this energetic charge. The new thought should evoke feelings of empowerment, strength or ease. Maybe it is 'settled' or 'peace'. Or a longer phrase of kindness, such as, 'May I trust in the unfolding of my life'. Repeat this thought like a mantra; you might write it down somewhere you can see it. Sometimes I repeat words with the cadence of my steps during everyday activities, in the grocery store or on the short walk from my car into the building where I work, each step repeating my word: 'trust', 'trust', 'trust'.

Spiritual Soul Work

Lori Dechar writes in *Alchemy of Inner Work* that Yi is the spirit that sings the heart's song into the world. In Chapter 1, you were asked to listen to what that song is. Working with the liver in Chapter 2, you were asked what singing it would look like, and the plan of where and when you are going to sing. Now, the spleen asks you to trust your song enough to sing it proudly into all facets of your life. In other words, the Yi is the doing part, the follow-through.

Again, following your Tao is about how your heart's authenticity comes alive in your day-to-day actions. For someone in their first half of life, this might look like committing to a project, a vocation or creating something new. In the second half, this might look like committing to a way of being in the world that brings the most joy. In either case, what are the actionable steps to start to live that most authentic expression? Because the spleen gets overwhelmed with thinking, writing down your thoughts in a journal can help organize them, so you can discern which ones mirror your intentions. Along with journalling, one of the most practical ways you can nourish the Yi is to write small and manageable to-do list. Writing a list is like emptying the mind of all of the 'I need to do', 'I really should do that', 'I am worried about' or 'I don't know what to do about' thoughts. It helps organize everything in the mind and propels you into action.

It is important when writing a to-do list that the steps are bite-sized. For example, do not write down something like 'Write a book'. Instead, get granular. Maybe write 'Text friend who wrote a book last year'. Breaking down a large intention into small tasks shows the mind that there has been movement towards what you want to manifest. After completing one item on your list, take a moment to celebrate before moving on to the next task.

Reflecting on your motivation and heart's intentions daily can help to ground them into your life. In many spiritual traditions, chanting and mantras were recited to hardwire intention – to set the heart's compass in the right direction. The voice tone of the Yi is the song, so physically singing helps to nourish the stomach and spleen on a spiritual level. If you don't like to sing, writing down your heart's deeper motivation and placing it somewhere visible can help remind you over and over again where you are going and what matters.

EXERCISE
CREATING YOUR TRUTH VOW

This exercise is meant to be a living enquiry, and always requires revision as you grow more and more into your authenticity. It can be done seated or standing.

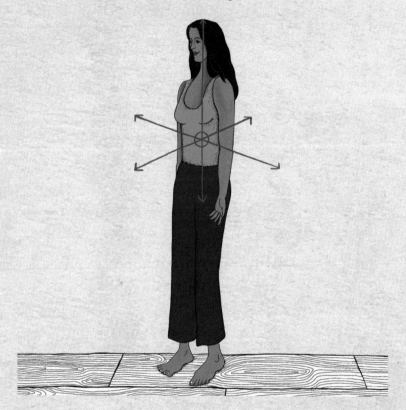

1 Take a few moments to find the vertical central energetic pole of your body that runs from the perineum to the crown of the head. Imagine this centre axis is like the earth's axis, staying steady. Take a few breaths, concentrating on this central axis that runs up and down.

GROUND OF INTENTION

2 Next, sense another axis that runs halfway between your perineum and crown horizontally, through the very centre of your torso. This line should be at about the level of your navel, or just above, around your solar plexus and below your heart.

3 Now, see if you can find the centre of your centre, where those two lines intersect. Breathe deeply here for a few moments. Notice any physical sensations you experience.

4 As you rest your attention at your centre, ask yourself the following questions:
   What is the guiding motivation behind all of my actions?'
   What is the guiding motivation behind all my actions?
   What does my heart want to devote itself to?
   What legacy do I want to leave behind?

Choose one word or, at most, a short phrase. Some examples could be 'authenticity', 'connection', 'love'. True intentions are motivated by benevolence and compassion, and are of service to the welfare of self and other. You might also feel a sense of expansion around the heart when you say that intention internally.

5 Next, reflect on one small action or micro-action that is devoted to that vow. Pick three small actionable steps to take towards it. Write these down, and follow through on one of them today.

6 Take the time to celebrate that intention, and notice how it feels to act in accordance with the truth of your heart.

CHAPTER 4
Holding On and Letting Go

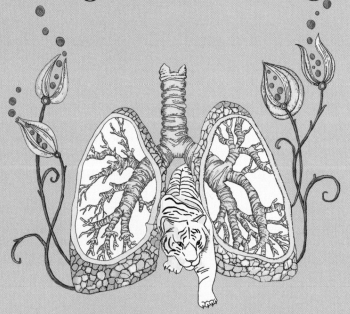

Spirit lessons from the
lungs and large intestine

'To live in this world, you must be able to do three
things: to love what is mortal; to hold it against your
bones knowing your own life depends on it; and,
when the time comes to let it go, to let it go.'

Mary Oliver

The stones sit silently by the lakeside, their pyrite flakes flash like coins against the evening sun. Glittering like precious gemstones, I pick one up and examine its shine. I put it in my pocket for safekeeping and continue to comb the beach. Each stone that catches my eye looks more beautiful than the last: pristine minerals sparkling like condensed starlight – the beauty of time and pressure. My pockets fill as I continue collecting stones, eventually bulging against my thighs. A raven flies low above me, and the sound of her wings lifts me from my trance. I stop my pillage and place the stones on a log in the shade to inspect them. I am disenchanted to see that without sunlight they are just lustless, ordinary stones. Dang! I scoop my treasure back into my hands, and reach them into the sun to once again see them sparkle back at me. I smile. I take a breath. I realize they have less value in my pocket then they do here on this beach, in harmony with their home landscape, dazzling each evening under the sun. And I also wonder: is the value in the stone, or is it in the sunlight or in the pyrite shavings? Or is the value in my perception of beauty? What is it exactly that I want to hold on to? What would having these stones give me, other than keeping the memory of this warm summer day alive? I lift my eyes to appreciate my surroundings and the awe I feel towards this moment, the sun now dipping towards the horizon. I drop all but one stone of medium size and sheen. My pockets feel lighter as I hold the one stone close, in the centre of my palm, feeling the essence of the sun reflect the memory of this place into my hand.

Found in minerals, stones and the refined elements of the air you breathe, the metal phase and its associated organs – the lungs and large intestine – represent the contracting entropic force that squeezes everything down to the most refined aspects of what you value. Like autumn and the setting sun, the metal phase delivers endings – death, grief, compost. And yet, it is at the end of a play where you discover the moral of the story – the gift, the point, the purpose of the entire drama. Each breath has the potency to remind you that you are bound to this earth plane, that time here is finite and that your life will one day be distilled down to the most important thing, which usually has nothing to do with money or material possessions. The spirit of the lungs and large intestine teaches us the value of ordinary moments and, when placed under the sunlight of our presence, how to be in awe of life's deepest mysteries.

The lungs also hold the wisdom of your body – not only your intuition, but the pain that has crystallized there; scars hidden within your psyche. Working with the lung energy, you are invited into the dark labyrinth of the soma (see page 135) to mine the depths of your personal past and to find the treasure hidden within your human limitations. When the lungs and large intestine are balanced, you are connected to your embodied existence, your mortality and your values. You carry a sense of self-worth, not for anything you have accomplished, but for the simple fact that you are alive. You are able to meet grief and death with dignity, and can flow with the winds of sorrow without losing your appreciation for life. The lungs and large intestine urge you to hold close the things you love, while at the same time encouraging you to let go, to walk with lighter pockets, and to step in flow with your sunlit surroundings.

ASSOCIATIONS

Spirit: Po

Element: Metal

Yin organ: Lungs

Yang organ: Large intestine

Animal: White tiger

Season: Autumn

Colour: White

Direction: West

Voice tone: Cry

Sense: Smell

Negative emotion: Grief

Balanced emotion: Awe, wonder, appreciation of life

Physical function: Respiration, skin and the immune system

Energetic function: Holding on to life/animal instincts, courage

Spirit function: Letting go, distilling values, virtue and integrity

PHYSICAL FUNCTION
RESPIRATION, SKIN AND DEFENSIVE QI

The lungs are large spongy organs that take up much of the upper half of the torso. From a Western medical perspective, the lungs are the main organs that help you breathe, and that work ceaselessly removes other gases, such as carbon dioxide, from your body. This process of respiration takes place 12 to 20 times per minute. The right lung and the left lung are slightly different sizes, with the right lung being wider and having three lobes, and the left lung smaller with only two. The size difference is due to the placement of the heart and the liver.

From the Chinese medicine perspective, the lungs govern all respiratory functions, including breathing and the physical health of the lungs, larynx and nose. They also have a very important role in the creation and maintenance of the immune system. This is because the lungs help to create and circulate what is known as Wei qi, which is a specific kind of energy that acts as protective shield within and around the body, and is the first line of defence against external pathogens. In addition to the immune system, the lungs are responsible for the health of the skin, the opening and closing of pores and the growth of body hair. In fact, the skin in Chinese medicine is known as the 'third lung'. Many skin-related issues are usually an indicator of lung energy being stressed or compromised in some way.

The large intestine (or colon) is the yang organ counterpart to the lungs. In Chinese medicine, the large intestine serves a similar purpose to what it does in Western medicine, which is elimination. It aids in the movement of waste downwards, and acts as the final organ to filter nutrients before they are eliminated from the body as stools. It primarily helps the body absorb electrolytes, minerals and water, and then eliminates waste from the body.

ENERGETIC FUNCTION
HOLDING ON AND INSPIRATION

Breathing is a universal process that connects you with all other living organisms: every creature on this planet has the drive to breathe and the desire to survive. Before we delve into the specifics of the lungs' energetics, please take a moment to take a few slow, deep breaths. Pay particular attention to the inhale and the various sensations as the air passes from your nose to your lungs. Now, exhale completely and hold your breath at the bottom. Pause, and before inhaling again, feel the quality of energy that wants to initiate inspiration – feel for the irrepressible pull that wants to draw breath in. Even as you read my words, see if you can hold your breath long enough to feel your body wanting to gasp for air. Eventually, you will have to breathe in – it is impossible to not to. You might be able to hold your beath until you pass out, but once you become unconscious, the body will start breathing for you. This short exercise exemplifies the energetics of the lungs: the choiceless instinct to survive.

The involuntary impulse you just felt to breathe is known as the Po, and is the spirit of the lungs and large intestine. I am introducing the spirit of the lungs in the energetics section because of its impact on the dynamics of attachment – it is nearly impossible to discuss energetic function of the lungs without familiarizing yourself with the Po. The Po represents your animalistic instinct to fiercely hold on to life. While the liver asserts the becoming of your spirit into the world through its dreams, the lungs assert the survival of your physical body through its impulses.

It is helpful to understand that the Po doesn't belong to you, but rather is a spirit of the earth that enters your body when you take your first breath. Also known as the corporeal soul, the Po is what tethers you to your body and the relative laws of impermanence during your life. It gifts you the same instinctual drives as all other animals and creatures that live on this planet, so it isn't personal – even your dog and the birds chirping outside your window have Po. Since the Po is also related to the large intestine, the anus is considered the 'Po Men' or 'the door of the Po'. When you die, it is said the Po exits through the anus, descending back into the earth.

The Po is a yin spirit because it represents the body unconscious. Unlike the spirits of the Hun and the Yi, whose intelligence and capabilities develop over time, the Po is nearly fully developed at birth. You can see the Po at work in a newborn baby who instinctually crawls up to latch on to her mother's breast. No one has taught baby to do this: it is innate. And, just as the lungs take hold of the particles in the air you need to breathe, so too does the Po take hold of the people, places and resources you need to sustain your life.

When the Po cannot hold on to what it is attached to, such as in the case of loss of a loved one or a major life transition, the lung energy collapses and the qi becomes obstructed; it is no longer able to latch and release. This is why grief is the main emotion associated with the lungs, and this can throw the lung and large intestine energy off balance.

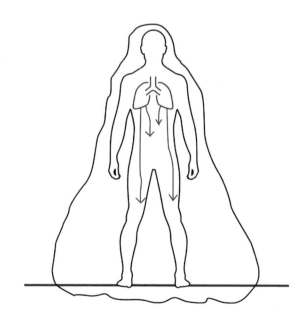

Touch and attachment – the doorway to intimacy

The Po is responsible for all physical sensations. When you touch something, the Po registers it as painful or pleasant, and either moves towards it or retracts from it in fear. The classic example would be placing your hand on a hot stove – you don't have to think about pulling it away from the painful sear of the heat. Without the Po to register pain and impulsively retract, we would damage our body unwittingly. All body sensations – getting a massage, petting your cat or scraping your knee – are registered by the Po. Another way to say this in simpler terms is the Po is the spirit that inhabits our soma, meaning the entire network of tissue that is alive with feeling. In Greek, 'soma' evolved to mean 'the body living in its wholeness'; the Po represents our animal body, and the totality of feeling of the personal unconscious.

In addition to warning the body of potential dangers, physical touch is a basic human need. It has been well documented that human babies can actually die from a lack of touch, or suffer from severe physical and cognitive developmental impairments without it. Physical touch is also required for proper development and functioning of the young of many species as they move into their adult phases.

The physical touch that the Po provides also opens the arena for intimacy. Touch, including sexual passion and pleasure, are all faculties of the Po. While the heart and the spirit of the Shen is what yearns for connection, the Po and the lungs are what make this connection possible through embodied experience. You feel connected to nature when feeling the sun against your skin or the sand between your toes. To feel a deep sense of connection, it is not simply enough to look out of a window or at a picture on your phone. You also feel more connected to those you love through physical touch. The feeling of pulling the one you love in close would not be possible without the Po. It is what clings on to what we need for survival: food, resources and of course LOVE. And while the heart (Shen) is what registers joy and connection, the Po offers us the sensations, touch and life force needed to actually receive it. Mortality is the doorway in which all love is received.

Psychologically, the energy of the lungs and large intestine is responsible for developing healthy attachment in relationships. Such attachment began when you were that little baby crawling up towards your mother's breast and has developed based on your relationship with your primary caregivers. Unlike gazelles born on the savanna who are able to run within a day, human babies are incredibly vulnerable for the first five years, and depend on guidance and nurturing for many years before being able to survive on their own. And so, at a very young age, the Po learns how to attach in order to satisfy its basic needs. If you didn't have parents who were attentive to your basic physical and emotional needs, this could lead to unhealthy attachment styles in adulthood, which are often triggered by close friends or romantic partners.

In spiritual communities there can be an over-emphasis on non-attachment and 'letting go' as a pathway to greater peace. And while renouncing human relationships can seem a lot more peaceful than the messiness of marriage, family or engaging with difficult people at work who trigger our attachment wounds, it is simply not possible to detach fully, nor is it a pathway to greater wellbeing. Our lungs want to attach to others in our community because it is part of our mammalian survival strategy.

Body memory

While the Po's capacities help us survive from birth, and include the basic instincts to breathe, crawl and latch, its patterns are further shaped as each person moves through life and learns how to best inhabit their body. The Po is what holds all unconscious memories, including basic physical abilities, such as walking, running and our ability to drive a car. It is what helps us perceive our body's physical position in space (proprioception) and the sensations within the body, such as feeling the heart beating, the lungs breathing or knowing when we are hungry (interoception). The Po is responsible for all physiological processes during childhood, and so our body is especially impressionable during this time. For example, if you performed gymnastics as a kid, your body potentially remembers how to do a cartwheel or a somersault over your lifetime without thinking about it. Just like you never forget how to ride a bike, the Po holds body memories that are automatic.

Courage

The Po is associated with the spirit animal of the white tiger, whose archetype exemplifies the lungs' instinct to protect and defend. In Chapter 1, we learned about the heart holding our soul's mandate, and how important it is to safeguard the Shen. It is noteworthy that the lungs physically surround the heart, and I like to think of them as the fourth, most distal heart protector.

The word 'courage' means 'with heart'. To act with our heart requires a modulation and titration of the Po's instinct with the guidance of the Shen's wisdom. When the Po is of service to the heart, our white tiger can stand with integrity and defend what we value with a combination of courageous ferocity, empathy and foresight. When the Po is taken over by a trauma memory, our instincts overtake the guidance of our heart, and our white tiger no longer acts out of courage but out of fear, which can lead to harming either self, or others. What helps the Po stay tethered to the heart is the Hun, the Shen's compassionate messenger. It is said that the that the Hun and the Po are always connected and dance together like a tiger and dragon. The Hun helps the Po titrate her instincts, and the Po offers the Hun physical power and intuition.

Remember, many of the Po's survival strategies were imprinted during childhood as body memory. It is through our breath that we can access the Hun's compassionate guidance, calm our impulses before acting, while at the same time, not suppress the intelligence that the Po offers. When working with past traumas and delving into body memories, a tremendous amount of courage is required, and our breath serves as the gateway to accessing it. If you reflect on a time when you had to summon bravery, you might notice yourself instinctively taking a deeper breath.

SPIRITUAL FUNCTION
LETTING GO

Take a moment to connect again with your breath. As you read, take a few deeper conscious breaths to connect directly with the energy of the lungs and their desire to 'hold' on to life. The next time you inhale deeply, hold your breath in. Feel the pressure build as you continue to hold. What is the quality of the energy behind your awaiting exhale? After exploring that for a few seconds, allow yourself to exhale and feel the sensation of release. Notice how your body might feel more relaxed, or more at ease in the support you are sitting or lying on.

If the energetic function of the lungs is about holding on to life, the spiritual function of the lungs is about letting go of life. While it is necessary to hold on to what we love and the things we need survive, it is equally important to let go of these very things in order to flow with the rhythm and seasons of our Tao. The lungs teach us that nothing in the relative world stays static, and that time brings ageing, change and eventually death. You will only physically die once in your life, but you might experience several psychological 'deaths' throughout a lifetime – you are not the same persona you were in your teenage years as you are in your late fifties! Each season of your life requires letting go of old habits and patterns, relationships and even physical objects that keep us held within our old identities. The lungs help us to stay flexible and flow with those changes.

Distilling what we value

The metal phase the lungs are associated with represents the end of the cycle, where the essences of the season are processed and stored. To make metal something of use and value requires refining through heat, distillation and pressure to remove non-metal elements. The downward pull of metal takes away what is no longer useful so that what is valuable can be extracted and appreciated.

When we think of metal in the process of respiration, every breath is a distillation of the pure from the impure – an opening to what is needed and a falling away of what is not. This distillation happens in every breath, the lungs miraculously extracting exactly what is needed from the air for our body to survive. This also happens in the large intestine in the process of digesting food, where the large intestine extracts electrolytes and minerals before finally releasing waste as excrement.

When I use the term 'let it go', I am not talking about the denial of life and I am also not talking about bypassing what is hard or difficult. The letting go that the lungs and large intestine gift us is the natural shedding of what is no longer needed, so that what is precious can be revealed. The paradox is that when we learn to let go, we start to refine our Tao more and more.

For instance, let's suppose there was a period in your life when you experienced social anxiety and depression. After discussing this with your therapist, you decided to start attending a weekly gathering with your colleagues on Friday nights at a local pub. By going out and socializing, your mood improved, and you felt more connected to your community. As time passed, you started reading more and listening to podcasts on wellbeing about how to maintain this positive life trajectory. You began prioritizing your health and made changes to your diet and exercise routine. Feeling better each day, you made the choice to join a running group that meets on Saturday mornings and found a new community there, which made you feel even more excited about your new life path. As time passed, you noticed that staying up late and drinking on Friday nights with your colleagues started impacting your ability to participate fully in the Saturday morning group. You also started to notice that you have less in common with your colleagues, who had little interest in the new things you were exploring. You found yourself at a crossroads: do you let go of the Friday night ritual or do you sacrifice the running group? There is no right answer to this question, and I think the real question here is: do you really value the community at the pub? Or do you value the running group and what living a life of health brings? Or is it both?

What I want to emphasize here is that the patterns that we are letting go of may not be inherently 'bad', just outdated. There are numerous instances where old routines and friendships fade away, usually after significant transition such as having children, starting a new job or making major changes in our lives. Just like a snake who has to shed its skin as it grows, we are asked to shed old ways of being that no longer work for the frequency that we wish to embody. Sometimes, this distillation process can be challenging and can require deep reflection, and even result in feelings of grief. Perhaps the hardest endings happen within relationships, but smaller endings happen all the time: the yoga class you once resonated with, the TV show you used to watch – we are always refining our values and how we want to spend our time. The lungs teach us that this is absolutely OK!

Death and grief

The lungs are teaching us through these many mini deaths how to approach our ultimate death with ease and grace. The Po, being a yin spirit, reminds us that we are not earthbound, and that everything we enjoy in life is impermanent. We are reminded of this by the constant flow of our breath, and the grief we feel after loved one's pass.

Grief happens when love bumps up against life's non-negotiables, when the lungs want to hold on but can't. Loss is the letting go that is not our choice, and the void we are thrust into because of it. Grief is the witnessing of sorrow and tragedy and, at the same time, in its healthy expression, it encourages us to still see the beauty in life. It is possibly one of the hardest teachers of the human experience, and no one who lives into their old age will avoid experiences of it. While grief is listed as one of the five 'negative' emotions in Chinese medicine, it is an unavoidable part of being alive. Grief, death and impermanence are part of the spiritual path. They urge us to wake up and to live fiercely with presence. It is just because our time is limited that we are forced to evaluate what we value and how we want to live. Without grief, life would not carry the same preciousness or poignancy.

The ultimate act of letting go is facing our own death. Tara Brach, a Buddhist teacher and psychologist, shares a story about a close friend of hers who works at a hospice, sitting with individuals who are nearing the end of their lives. One afternoon, he sat with an elderly woman who had been receiving care for some time and was ready to pass away. She expressed to him that she was ready to die but didn't know how. 'Everyone keeps telling me that I just need to let go, but I don't know how. Do you?' She looked eagerly to him. He smiled and took her hand in response, and squeezed it and then let it go, and squeezed it and let it go. 'It's like that,' he said. Nurses entered the room to check her vital signs, measure her blood pressure and administer medications. As they worked, the old woman held his hand and practised the squeezing and releasing motion. 'I think I understand now,' she said to him. The following day, she died. What resonates with me in this story is that letting go is truly that: a release. While it occurs within the mind, it also necessitates a physical surrender. Our bodies hold on tightly to life due to fear. The spiritual journey of letting go involves embracing the flow of this release into the greater rhythm of life.

'Grief and love are sisters ...
their kinship reminds us that there is
no love that does not contain loss and
no loss that is not a reminder of the love
we carry for what we once held close.'

Francis Weller,
*The Wild Edge of
Sorrow* (2015)

WHERE YOU GET STUCK
BODY PAIN, AUTOIMMUNE DISORDERS AND TRAUMA

As you have learned so far, the Po governs automatic body memories that aid in our functioning and survival. This frees up space in our mind for other more conscious processes, such as imagination and thought. Unfortunately, the Po is also shaped by negative body memories, especially those from childhood. In fact, any degree of trauma, including neglect or bullying, or even smaller everyday traumas, will be stored memories in the body. The Po learns from these experiences and, like a soldier on guard, learns how to brace itself against these possible threats. Again, these body memories are different to conscious memories, so we might not be aware of how they are still operating within us. If you were asked to sing in your Grade One music class, for example, but then were ostracized for having a bad singing voice, your Po learned it was unsafe to sing. You might still unconsciously hold or block that area of your body and have extreme anxiety of singing in front of others.

The lungs and large intestine also relate to the primal sense of smell, which is a common association that can be linked to memory. For instance, if your mother was an alcoholic whose drink of choice was white wine, you might be triggered by the smell of chardonnay at a Christmas party, and experience an onset of increased heart rate, anxiety or a panic attack, or other emotions indicating a feeling of being unsafe. The Po established a connection early in your life equating white wine with danger, which helped you to survive, and now, even though white wine poses no physical threat, the Po soul is stuck in that pattern.

Much of the time, traumatic body memories remain hidden in the unconscious until they show themselves as a body pain or nervous response. Think back to the heart chapter where you learned about shock and trauma. When trauma occurs, the little red bird of the heart flies back up to heaven where it is safe. The Po – the white tiger – is left to defend the physical body without guidance from the conscious mind. In extreme cases, where the Shen vacates the body completely, there might not be a conscious memory of the trauma at all. Instead, it is locked away within the body's unconscious. As we start to bring the Shen back home into the body, through qigong, breathwork and meditation practices, memories that are locked in the personal unconscious can start to reveal themselves.

You might be wondering, what is the point of digging up the past? Why is it worth getting into past grievances? The point is to help disarm the white tiger's outdated survival strategies, which can be especially problematic when the defences are tightened against the self. Often, children inadvertently blame themselves for the traumatic events they experienced. These belief systems then become concealed within the unconscious mind and develop into inner 'demons', which include addictions, violent outbursts, insecure attachment patterns and chronic pain. In more severe cases, the white tiger can wreak havoc on our immune system, leading to autoimmune disorders where the immune system mistakenly attacks its own the body. Interestingly, there have been numerous correlations between autoimmune disorders and early childhood trauma, with certain therapies, including eye movement desensitization and reprocessing (EDMR) and internal family systems (IFS) helping to reduce pain.

When the Po is left to its own devices, that is if our Shen and Hun remain dissociated from the body, its impulses keep us stuck in pleasure-seeking and pain-avoidance patterns. From a medical qigong perspective, this is how addictions, anxiety disorders and other severe mental health disorders happen. In Chinese medicine, it is said all virtues come from the Shen and the Hun, while all 'demons' come from the Po. The impulses cannot be abandoned by the 'higher', more conscious-thought processes, and our spiritual 'work' is about re-associating the conscious mind with the unconscious mind.

Opening the doorway to the past is painful, but it is the only way to rejoin the conscious mind with the unconscious – bringing the shadows to light and disarming our outdated survival strategies. To be clear, trauma does not have to be extreme: small traumas, such as how we were not seen or heard as a child or the way a sibling treated us, can have an impact on the quality of our body and its demons in our adult life.

Because the lungs relate to preciousness and values, low self-worth is a classic sign of a Po disturbance. This manifests in various ways, one of which is a constant need to prove oneself or equating personal value with accomplishments in life. When we rely on external validation from friends, partners or the number of followers we have on social media to determine our value, it can indicate a lack of self-worth.

Additionally, low self-worth can affect our intimate relationships through unhealthy attachment styles. Anxiously attaching oneself and displaying clingy behaviour out of fear that a partner will leave is a common manifestation. This fear stems from the belief that one is not enough or that their partner will never be enough. On the other hand, some individuals may avoid intimacy altogether due to similar fears or doubts about their own worthiness.

In contrast, individuals with high self-worth have a stronger sense of intrinsic value, which is not dependent on external validation or achievements. They are less likely to seek constant reassurance and are able to maintain healthier attachment styles in their relationships. Developing and nurturing a healthy sense of self-worth is crucial for overall wellbeing. It involves challenging and examining the unconscious belief systems we carry, questioning the cultural messaging we have internalized, and shifting our focus towards internal validation rather than external sources. This process allows us to embrace our worthiness and establish more fulfilling and authentic connections with both ourselves and others.

Denying fate

Whether or not you believe in 'fate', I use the word here to point to all the things in life that are out of our control, such as who our parents are, where we were born, our past traumas, loss and, ultimately, death. The lungs and large intestine teach us that grief is a universal rite of passage which, when confronted directly, leads to greater flexibility and compassion.

In a culture that denies death collectively – viewing it as a medical failure rather than a metaphysical event – denial can block the lungs' natural capacity for flexibility and acceptance. Interestingly, denial is the first stage of grief that we have to move through, but if we stay in it, it keeps us fighting with our fate, ironically distancing us from our destiny (our Tao).

If we run from our fate and the grief it stirs up, we become hardened by it. The difficulties we avoid eventually find us within the pain of our body armour and result in disease. Running from challenging circumstances causes the body to 'clench', restricting our qi flow and leading to illness. Moreover, denying reality puts us in a state of half-presence. Like only partially inhaling due to fear of exhaling, the lungs become inflexible and stiff. So, in our attempt to escape fate, we ironically escape life.

We live in a culture that seeks pleasure and avoids pain, one that hides from death and difficulty. I once worked at a yoga studio where the throw pillows in the entrance lounge read, 'Breathe in the good, breathe out the bad'. This is precisely the opposite of what the lungs are trying to teach us! The courage that the lungs give us is the capacity for us to bear witness to the 'bad'. When a loved one dies, we should not deny the pain; instead, it needs to be processed and witnessed with care – something that takes time and a lot of support. The road from denial to acceptance can be a long one, but, eventually, the more we can witness and hold ourselves in compassion, the closer we get to acceptance.

Symptoms

Take a look at the symptoms opposite, which can arise when lung and large intestine energy are thrown off. If you notice any of these themes in your life, especially if you experience at least one symptom in each category, it might indicate that these organs need some love!

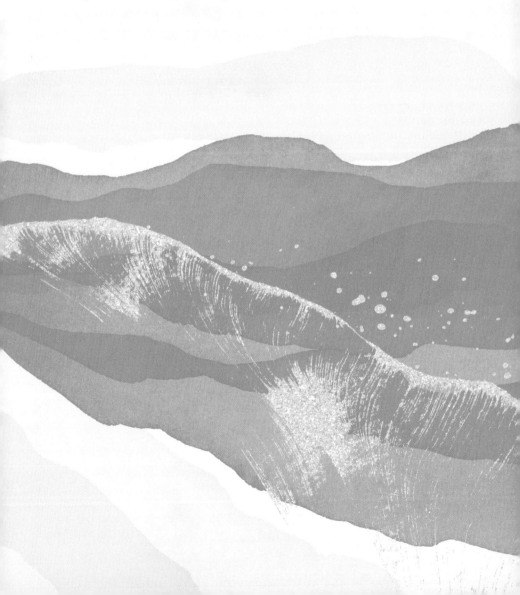

PHYSICAL

- ❋ respiratory issues
- ❋ skin disorders
- ❋ weak immune system
- ❋ auto-immune disorders
- ❋ chronic pain
- ❋ numbness (inability to feel)
- ❋ inflammatory bowel diseases

ENERGETIC

- ❋ inability to process grief
- ❋ stuck in denial/avoidance
- ❋ pleasure-seeking behaviours
- ❋ insecure attachment patterns in relationships
- ❋ inability to hold and cherish what is valuable in life

SPIRITUAL

- ❋ inability to let go of what is no longer valuable
- ❋ holding on to the past and clinging to past identities
- ❋ low self-worth
- ❋ inability to know what you value
- ❋ loss of dignity and integrity, being 'taken over' by your impulses

SOUL WORK
FROM IMPULSIVITY TO INTEGRITY

The soul work for the lungs requires you to tend to your body's animalistic needs (survival, social and sensual). The lungs invite you to hold what you love close, and at the same time learn how to let go when the time is right. The lungs ask you to honour grief as a process during times of loss or major life change.

Physical Soul Work

For physical soul work for the lungs, it is important to activate the breath and engage in activities that promote embodiment. Breathing through your nose, particularly at night, can benefit your lungs. If you tend to breathe through your mouth, using a neti pot or nasal spray can aid breathing through the nose. Practising breath-awareness meditation, focusing on the sensations of the breath at the nose and when entering the lungs, can help connect your conscious mind (Shen and Hun) with the typically involuntary act of breathing. Any form of breathwork is beneficial for the lungs, but I recommend you work with a skilled practitioner for more vigorous breathing exercises.

Activities such as yoga, qigong and other movement practices that embody animal-like movements can be helpful for the Po. The lungs often respond well to primal movements, such as dancing, shaking, stretching and walking in natural landscapes. It may sound simple, but regularly checking in with your body throughout the day can nourish the Po. Just like responding to thirst by drinking water, or standing up and stretching after sitting at work, listening to your body's impulses to care for your animal body – much like you would care for your pets – can support wellbeing!

Since the lungs are connected to all bodily sensations, becoming more sensual throughout the day can nourish lung energy. This involves not only embracing healthy sexuality and intimate touch from loved ones, but also engaging with activities that stimulate the senses, like burning incense, diffusing essential oils or listening to beautiful music.

EXERCISE
ACUPRESSURE LI-14 'TIGER'S MOUTH'

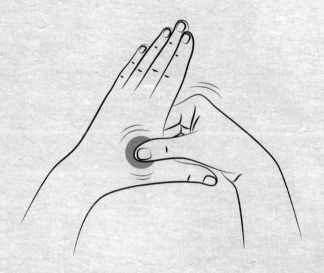

LI-4 (Large Intestine 4) is an energy point along the large intestine channel that is easy to stimulate and very powerful for clearing qi stagnation in the lungs. The point is called He Gu or Hu Kou, meaning either 'joining valley' or 'tiger's mouth'. This point is also effective for boosting the immune system, relieving constipation and diarrhoea, clearing headaches and reducing sinus and body pain.

Please note: this point should not be used while pregnant because it encourages the downward flow of qi and can induce labour.

1 Find the point. The LI-4 is in the soft hollow beyond the intersection of your thumb and index finger bones. This area is typically slightly sore, especially when it's in need of attention.

2 Stimulate the point. Use gentle to moderate pressure in small circular motions in the area for a few minutes. If you are using this point for acute sinus or body pain, you can massage it throughout the day. Make sure you stimulate both sides evenly. Use the acupressure exercise as a way of connecting to your body.

3 You can also activate the point by applying diluted essential oils on the skin using a cotton swab. Cypress, clary sage, rosemary, peppermint or eucalyptus oils all relate to the metal phase and lung/large intestine energy.

Energetic Soul Work

On an energetic level, soul work for the lungs and large intestine involves becoming more attuned to your body's impulses. This includes recognizing not only physical needs, such as hunger, thirst and the need for rest, but also emotional needs and attachment triggers. If, for example, you become anxious when your partner doesn't reply to your texts, you could be noticing the emergence of the 'white tiger' of the Po. Ask yourself what the tiger is afraid of. What might it want or need? Tending to your animal body rather than fighting against it is a crucial first step in disarming inner demons.

This all being said, there is a thin line between taking care of your body's needs and following every impulse. It is essential that the Hun (your conscience) be tethered to your body, so that the energy of the impulse is taken care of; so it doesn't run wild and cause harm to yourself or others through impulse behaviour, overindulgence or violence. Part of the soul work for the lungs is noticing impulse, relating to it, and then consciously deciding what is needed.

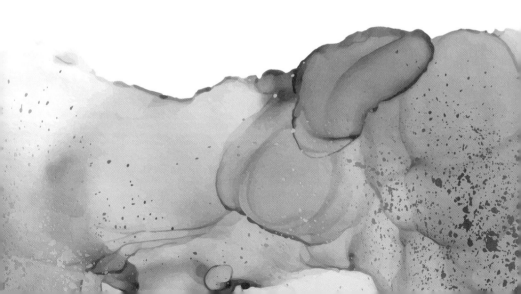

EXERCISE
FEEDING YOUR WHITE TIGER

This practice is helpful when strong emotions have been triggered surrounding attachments; for example, if your partner or friend triggers you, or if you feel jealous or guilty or ashamed. You can also use this exercise to address any chronic pain or inflammation in the body that you feel frustrated towards.

1 Find a comfortable place to sit or lie down. Take a moment to survey the room or area you are in by looking all around, including up and down. Make sure to move your neck and eyes, as this helps to activate your autonomic nervous system, signalling to yourself that you are safe.

2 Once you feel comfortable, gently close your eyes. Take three deep, full breaths, counting to five on each inhale and exhale.

3 Now, take a moment to bring to mind the trigger and explore how it makes you feel in your body. If it involves physical pain, locate that sensation within your body.

What is the shape, colour, texture and size of the energy associated with the trigger?
Does the energy exhibit any movement?
What does the energy say to you, and in what tone of voice?

4 See if you can foster curiosity towards the sensation, allowing it to express itself. Sometimes it is hard to hold our pain with curiosity and acceptance because our natural tendency is to fight with it. If you feel a strong emotion towards your pain, notice that emotional response in your body. For example, you might feel frustration towards your rheumatoid arthritis. Work with the frustration first.

5 If the emotional response becomes overwhelming or brings up too many memories, open your eyes, look around the room, feel into your hands and feet and kindly ask it to slow down and give you some space.

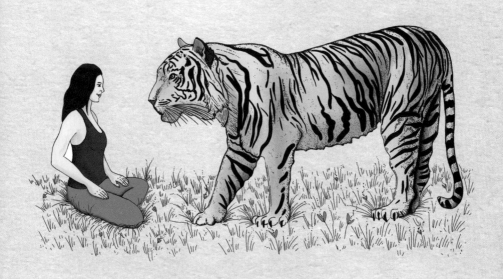

6 Now imagine the energy exiting through a small opening beneath your collarbones, transforming into a white tiger that now sits in front of you. See this tiger as a protective force and an ally that has become temporarily misplaced. Ask the tiger:

What are you protecting me from?
What do you need to feel okay?
Do you have any messages for me?

7 If the tiger appears particularly fierce, begin deepening your breath. Envision a radiant white light at the centre of your chest. As you breathe in, 'take in' the tiger's fears, worries and pain, genuinely acknowledging them. As you exhale, feel that white light radiating into your lungs and towards the white tiger, calming her.

8 Repeat this deep breathing with the white light for as long as necessary until the white tiger becomes calm. If you have a physical pain in your body, send that white light to the pain. The most important thing is to deeply witness and acknowledge the pattern, not fight with it, and at the same time to not act from it.

9 Before opening your eyes, ask the white tiger what it is asking of you. Is there something you can do in your daily life to remind her that you are safe?

10 If you like, journal what came up, whether it was a memory, an insight or simply a body 'felt sense'.

Spiritual Soul Work

The spiritual level of soul work for the lungs and large intestine involves supporting the processes of 'letting go'. I have identified a few different flavours of letting go, which include renunciation, hard decisions at the crossroads and navigating loss and grief. As you read through these, see which are most relevant to your life in the season you are in.

Renunciation

Renunciation is a core monastic practice that usually involves abandoning actions such as violence towards oneself and others, stealing, lying, slander and gossip. The etymology of the word renunciation means 'to protest against'. When we let go of patterns that harm ourselves and others, we are 'protesting against' habitual energies that keep us from living our Tao. It is hard to know our Tao if we don't know peace, and it is hard to know peace if we are engaging in violence towards self or other.

For many of us, when we think of renunciation, we think of 'having' to give up something. But the renunciation that supports the lungs is not always about denying the body the things it enjoys, rather, it is about letting go of the heavy burdens that cause suffering.

An obvious example of what causes harm is violence towards others, and some less obvious examples are negative self-talk and gossip. In medical qigong, it is believed that when you lie or act out of integrity it creates holes in the Wei qi (protective energy field), lowering your immune system and making you more vulnerable to energies around you. Whether or not you believe in this, gossip and violence are low vibrational activities that usually make us feel bad.

Take a moment to reflect. What are the boulders you pick up unnecessarily? What would feel good (in the long run) to put down?

Hard decisions at the crossroads

Once you let go of what is causing harm, the messages of your heart will become clear, and you can further distil what you value. This distillation starts to express itself as decisions towards enacting those values; because while there are aspects of life that are fated (what you can't control), there are many things that you can. Every decision you make is a crossroad between holding on to one thing and letting go of another.

If you are truly committed to living authentically, there may come a time where you find yourself at a major crossroads where, at a deep level, you know letting go is necessary – this is a process that demands tremendous courage. Some examples of this could be break-ups or divorce, friendships ending, saying 'No' to a marriage proposal, moving across the country or quitting your job. These big 'letting go' moments can bring about huge transformations on the level of the soul. If you are going through one of these moments, it is important to seek support from those who are open to your growth, like a trusted friend or therapist, and remember that the heart (the Shen) will be your 'truest' advisor.

Aside from these big changes, you can live in accordance with your values in small ways. How we spend our time and money is a direct reflection of our values, so continually re-evaluating this is the soul work of the lungs; be this thinking about the TV shows you watch, the friends you spend your time with or what you buy at the grocery store.

Take a few moments to reflect on what you value. Maybe even take the time to write down your top five. Are you spending your resources, namely your time and money, on those things? Are there any big things you need to let go of so you can walk more fully into your authentic expression?

Navigating grief

Lastly, the lungs and large intestine ask you to navigate grief consciously and courageously. Depending on the extent of your loss, this could be a long process and might involve journalling, support groups and therapy, as well as meaningful rituals or ceremonies.

Giving grief a place to be expressed is especially important so that its energy has somewhere to flow. Maybe it is a creative project, such as painting, writing or music, or maybe it is a new physical activity, such as dance or kickboxing. It is important not to always dive into the very depths of your grief, but rather titrate it, spending time doing things that bring joy, and spending time feeling into the loss and allowing yourself to shed the necessary tears. Engaging in qigong practices that support the lungs will be especially helpful at this, as well as the meditation practices, such as the one described below.

"If you are truly committed to living authentically, there may come a time where you find yourself at a major crossroad where, at a deep level, you know letting go is necessary"

EXERCISE
EMBODYING LETTING GO

This exercise is a variation of progressive muscle relaxation combined with the breath-retention techniques used in qigong. It also incorporates the healing sound for the lungs, which resembles the hissing sound of a snake, 'ssss'. The purpose of this practice is to help the Po relax and to cultivate the quality of letting go. You can do this exercise at any time during the day or, if you have trouble falling asleep, you can do it before bed.

* Note: You will be taking multiple small sips of breath in without exhaling, so make sure to only inhale a small amount of breath at a time.

1 To begin, find a comfortable lying-down position on a flat surface, such as the floor or a bed.

2 Once comfortable, direct your attention towards your feet. Inhale a small, gentle sip of breath and tighten your feet, squeezing you toes towards your heels.

3 Take another small sip of breath in and tighten your legs and buttocks.

4 Sip in again and tighten your torso, arms and hands. Make tight fists and slightly flex your biceps.

5 Take in a bit more breath and tighten your facial muscles.

6 Finally, take another breath, inhaling fully, and tighten your entire body. Hold this tension for a moment.

7 Now, exhale slowly through your mouth, making the sound 'sssssss', as if you're gradually deflating a balloon. Relax your face, torso, fists, buttocks, legs and feet (in that order, top to bottom).

8 Take a few natural deep breaths, allowing your body to sink. Repeat this process for a total of three rounds and pay attention to how you feel.

CHAPTER 5
From Fear to Faith

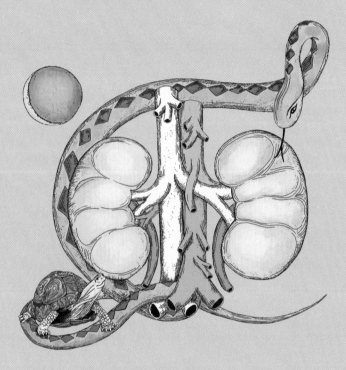

Spirit lessons from the
kidneys and bladder

'My kidneys instruct me in the night season.'

The Bible, Psalm 16, verse 7

My cross-country skis glide along the icy terrain, the 'swish, swish' sound muffled by my hat, hood and scarf. The Canadian winters, so fiercely cold, cause every bit of life to retract into hiding, leaving the landscape silent. Even the snow that blows off the tree branches floats noiselessly to the forest floor, glimmering fat flakes with no witness but my eyes. As the trees and animals sleep peacefully under the snow, I move through the white muted landscape in awe of the purity of nature's pause. I am amazed that in just a few months these same meadows will be teaming with wildflowers, bugs and songbirds – it hardly seems possible. The icy wind bites my face as I slide along an almost unmarked track and wonder how anything could stay alive through this deep dark freeze. I reach a clearing where the snow has blown into a dune, with a defined ridge that reaches the height of my shoulders. After a moment admiring its prestige, I pop off my skis, turn around, and put my arms out to the sides, like Jesus on the cross. I let my body fall back into the bank and land with a soft 'thunk'. I close my eyes. Dark, still and so, so quiet. I fall into the silence like quicksand, hearing nothing but the faint sound of my own heartbeat, amplified by the layers wrapped round my head. I allow myself to be held like a foetus cocooned within the snowbank – the silence nourishing my inner ears, and the dormant landscape welcoming me under her winter quilt of respite. I stay in my frozen La-Z-Boy for a long time, eyes closed, like a hibernating bear, my back and bones fully supported, until I feel the cold of the snow start to leach from the bank through my snowpants. Eventually, I emerge from the dune and dust myself off, feeling refreshed and inspired by nature's dormancy and the power she is able to generate through simply resting.

Being the most yin of all the organs, the kidney and bladder and associated season of winter call us to step in harmony with a wiser, more natural rhythm. While the lungs teach us to let go to the process of decay and death, the kidneys teach us to patiently wait in the realm of the unknown – in the silent space after death but before birth. Just as I discovered that day in the snow, a life that is energetically sustainable requires time for our bones to rest and ears to listen. Rest is a necessary part of gestation. Just as sap sinks to the roots and bears retreat to their dens to conserve their qi, the kidneys encourage us to retreat when conditions are frigid and our efforts to be 'productive' are futile. The kidneys inspire faith in life's divine timing, encouraging us to lean back into our naturalness instead of unnecessarily pushing or forcing something when the energy isn't there. As we become more attuned to our kidneys, bladder and the spirit of the water element, we start to feel more comfortable in this liminal space and can wait there until we sense the pulse of our Tao moving us into action.

The kidneys, bladder and the water phase are dual in nature, because although they teach us how to rest, in doing so they generate a tremendous amount of power. As a shape-shifter, water can both freeze and thaw, boil and steam. While it is soft, it has the power to move rocks and shape landscapes. When you listen deeply to your kidneys, you listen directly to the force of creation that knows exactly the right time to act and the right time to rest – like the sap rising from the roots, the bear waking from hibernation, and the seed that knows just when to sprout.

The kidneys teach you that the more you align with your Tao, the more you will 'plug in' to a greater energy source that gives you the horsepower needed to physically embody it – without forcing or striving. The kidneys remind us that our Tao is not a race to the finish line, and most of the time life does not always happen in the way, shape or form that we have planned. And while the kidneys deplete in their physical 'essence' with each passing year, they grow with wisdom each time you surrender into the sacred listening pause.

ASSOCIATIONS

Spirit: Zhi

Element: Water

Yin organ: Kidneys

Yang organ: Bladder

Animal: Tortoise and snake

Season: Winter

Colour: Blue

Direction: North

Voice tone: Groan

Negative emotion: Fear

Balanced emotion: Faith

Physical function: Storage of essence (jing), governance of water, regulates bone health, hearing, reproduction, brain health and short-term memory

Energetic function: Focus, skilful use of resources, risk assessment

Spirit function: Inner awareness and self-understanding, aligned will, wisdom, connection to ancestors

PHYSICAL FUNCTION
THE FOUNDATION OF OUR VITALITY

The kidneys are bean-shaped organs that sit on either side of your spine at about the height of your mid-back, extending from the third lumbar disc to about the thirteenth thoracic disk. The left kidney sits slightly higher than the right, due to the placement of the liver. The average kidney is about the size of a fist, 10–15 cm (4–6 in) long. In Western medicine, the kidneys are responsible for filtering waste products and excess fluid from your system, and for maintaining the proper balance of water, salts and minerals in your blood. The kidneys also produce hormones that help to control blood pressure, stimulate the production of blood cells and promote the health and strength of the bones.

From the perspective of Chinese medicine, the kidneys are different to the other yin organs because they are foundational for all yin and yang energies in the body: the left kidney being more yin, and right kidney more yang. The yin of the kidneys nourishes the liver, heart and lungs, ruling the cycle of birth, growth, maturation and water metabolism, while the yang of the kidney relates to the function of heating and moving qi, and this primary motivating force begins all the body's physiological processes. I like to think of the kidneys as the batteries of our physical body, because without them and their positive (yang) and negative (yin) charge, no other organ system would be able to function.

The kidneys play a particularly important role in our physical health and energy levels because they store a substance called *jing*. *Jing* is what qi (energy) is made of and forms the foundation of our physical vitality. It is also known as 'prenatal qi' and is inherited from our parents. Each person is born with a certain amount of *jing*, which depletes as one ages. A lot of qigong and Chinese medicine practices were designed to help conserve *jing*, to aid in a graceful ageing process. *Jing* determines our genetic constitution and is responsible for fertility, reproduction, growth, development and ageing. Anything that is considered genetic or hereditary in modern terms can be attributed to the kidneys. The kidneys determine our physical blueprint, including our height, hair and skin colour, and susceptibility to diseases.

In addition to regulating water metabolism and producing hormones, the kidneys also govern the 'sea of marrow' which affects the health of our bones, bone marrow, spinal fluid and brain. Therefore, the health of the entire skeleton – the knees, spine and the proper functioning of the brain – relies on the kidneys. They also nourish the essences responsible for hair growth, so hair loss and greying hair are also attributed to kidney energy. The kidneys are particularly linked to the brain function of short-term, working memory and the faculty of hearing and the physical health of the ears, all functions that tend to decline with age.

The bladder is a muscular sac in the pelvis, sitting just above and behind the pubic bone. It is connected to the kidneys through two tubes called ureters that deliver urine from the filtered fluid of the kidney. The bladder's flexible cavity is about the size of a pear when empty, expanding to hold up to 500 ml (1 pint) of fluid when full. The main function of the bladder from the perspective of both Western and Chinese medicine is to store and secrete urine from the body. However, in Chinese medicine, the bladder is more connected to the left kidney.

> "The kidneys teach you that the more you align with your Tao, the more you will 'plug in' to a greater energy source that gives you the horsepower needed to physically embody it."

ENERGETIC FUNCTION
SURVIVAL

As with the lungs, one of the primary energetic functions of the kidneys and bladder is survival. While the lungs help to signal the 'fight, flight and freeze' response through somatic memory, the kidneys provide the energy needed to actually run or fight.

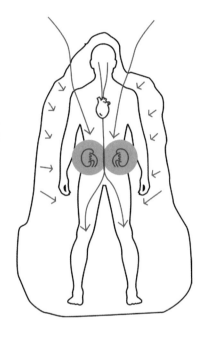

The kidneys are not only concerned with personal survival, but also that of your family and lineage. They give you the desire and drive to reproduce and to leave the legacy of your family line. Therefore, sexual drive and libido relate to healthy functioning kidneys.

The kidneys and bladder also relate to the primal emotion of fear, which is the emotion most closely linked with survival. When the body is afraid, the energy moves in and down the front of the body from the eyes to the groin, preparing it to flee, fight or freeze. The adrenal glands, which sit like little hats on top of the kidneys, are like the pilot light that, when activated, can give us a flood of extra energy from our reserves. Examples of this include a mother lifting a car to save her child or a small woman dragging her husband out of a burning building; the kidneys give us an energy 'boost' when we absolutely need it. Without fear our species would certainly not be alive, because it helps us avoid or escape life-threatening situations. In addition to extreme situations, the kidneys help us to mediate risk when it comes to our physical safety: they are what scans for possible hazards when we go skiing, for example, and helps us prepare and choose which items we put in our backpack when we go on a rock-climbing

FROM FEAR TO FAITH

trip. We need the kidneys to watch out for our physical wellbeing and the wellbeing of our family.

While fear can certainly be a problematic emotion when it becomes chronic, its energetic blueprint is not inherently bad. Remember back to the wood phase and the liver chapter – anger is the movement up and out, and which carries the similar energetic pattern of fierce compassion and the psychic energy needed to assert your plans and dreams. Similarly, the balanced movement of the kidneys and bladder, namely in and down, helps with heightened awareness in order to mediate risks and aid focused concentration and the motivation to act, as well as the ability to intelligently conserve resources. The key here is balancing these energies and working with them, rather than fighting with them or letting them run wild.

Heightened awareness

The kidneys possess an extraordinary ability to heighten our awareness, much like a vigilant young deer sensing a heartbeat from miles away. They hold a profound, innate understanding, similar to the wisdom possessed by birds when they build their nests or migrate south, or the knowing within our bones when weather changes. By tapping into the dark perceptive power of the kidneys, you are able to mediate risks appropriately – not solely based on logic, but on what feels right to your animal body. In listening to the kidneys' attentiveness, you know when it is safe to walk home late at night or if it is best to call a cab; or when to put a down payment on a house and when to walk away. The more you can learn to discern and trust this nervous awareness and what it is trying to tell you, the more fear can be a teacher and a guidepost, rather than a 'bad' energy you feel you need to rid yourself of.

Remembering

The kidneys and bladder are responsible for your ability to focus and concentrate through sustaining your short-term memory. Commonly known as 'working memory', the kidney energy is what maintains your attention on your intention. For example, let's say you got up from your kitchen table to go and change over the laundry. If your working memory is on point, you will get to the machine and complete the task. If it isn't, you might get part way there, start petting your cat, check your phone, straighten out the family photos on the wall and forget why you got up in the first place! This example highlights the relationship between the spirit of the stomach and spleen (Yi and intention) and the spirit of the kidneys and bladder (Zhi and will). You can have an intention, but unless there is energy to sustain the intention, the focus will be lacking to actually complete the task.

In the ancient texts of the *Huangdi Neijng*, it is said, 'When intent becomes permanent, we speak of will.' Will, or Zhi, refers to the spirit of the kidneys and the horsepower that our intention depends on. While the Yi formulates intentions from the heart, the Zhi provides the concentrated focus and memory needed for those intentions to manifest into actions. In doing so, our energy is not scattered, but is rather directed towards the activities, relationships and projects that matter most to us.

In Sanskrit, the word for mindfulness is *smriti*, which means 'to remember'. It is fascinating that both the heart and the kidneys – the most 'yang' organ and the most 'yin' organ – are connected to memory. Memory plays a crucial role in our spiritual journey because it is the faculty of mind that allows us to first contact, and then enact, our Tao. Being mindful means remembering our soul's purpose by accessing the long-term memory stored within our hearts – namely, why our spirits chose to inhabit a physical body on this planet – while also engaging in moment-to-moment remembrance by acting in alignment with those truths. While the heart provides us with glimpses of profound insights, if we fail to uphold this memory through our everyday actions (the memory of the kidneys), our Tao remains an idea in the clouds, rather than a path we consciously choose to walk. And on very practical levels, the short-term memory and focus of the kidneys allows us to complete mundane tasks, such as changing over the laundry, focusing on the book we are reading, or staying attentive to tasks at work!

Prepare and conserve

The kidneys and bladder motivate us to work, gather, prepare and conserve our resources. On a physical level, the kidneys store our most valuable resource: our energy and the time we have to live. Their energetic functioning prompts us to prepare and manage other essential resources, like time and money. It's important to note that the kidneys embody both yin and yang characteristics. They invite us to rest, reflect, meditate and conserve, while simultaneously providing us with the power and motivation to act.

The motivation to gather resources and plan ahead is undeniably necessary – we all need a roof over our heads and food in our bellies to sustain our lives. The bladder, as a flexible receptacle for storage, is closely tied to the concept of resource management. Much like a squirrel that stores nuts for the winter, the kidneys and bladder instil in us the foresight and drive to save resources, allowing us to navigate life with enough energy to live and thrive.

This drive to save and conserve becomes particularly pronounced before having a child, and mothers often start 'nesting' by gathering baby items and saving money to ensure a sufficient maternity leave. Similarly, we may also notice this drive to save and prepare for our children's future, such as by starting a bank account for their education, or when we start contemplating retirement in later years. In this context, a healthy amount of fear can be beneficial. If fear didn't exist, we might recklessly deplete our resources and be unprepared for less productive or more passive phases of life. Fear can motivate us to work hard and be mindful of conserving, ensuring we have the resources to enjoy relaxation during the quieter 'winter' phases of our lives. Therefore, a bit of fear in order to prepare will actually reduce stress.

Spiritual Function
SELF-UNDERSTANDING

Symbolic of the vast blue/black depths of the ocean, the kidneys serve as a portal through which we can explore the mysterious depths of our being. Unlike the heart and liver, which guide our outward perceptions and aspirations, the kidneys invite us to engage with the shadowy realm of understanding our soul and its story. By listening deeply to our dreams, noticing synchronicities and connecting their meaning to our life narrative, we uncover more profound layers of self-understanding.

This process can uncover both our deepest wounds and greatest gifts, some of which may have originated in our childhood or have been passed down through generations. When these wounds emerge from the darkness, they call for our attention, curiosity and care.

For example, a few years ago I started to notice a pattern in myself where I would work so hard that I burned out, needing to take a month off work to recover. Ironically, I had been teaching yoga, meditation and qigong since my early twenties, which focused on helping people to relax and prevent burnout. On a conscious level, I knew this pattern needed to stop, as it contradicted my own teachings, but despite that awareness, it continued to play out.

During one of my episodes of burnout, I had a vivid dream of an elk stag standing in a public bathroom shower, with its back hollowed out and blood streaming out from within the shower water. It was a disturbing image, and even more unsettling was the fact that in the dream my mother told me they had eaten the back of the elk for a family dinner. This dream image was embedded within me and instead of letting it fall back as a lost memory, I opened my awareness to it as a messenger. After that dream, it felt like I couldn't escape the presence of elk in my everyday life. They seemed to appear everywhere, from artwork to TV shows to my trips to the mountains. A few weeks later, I had a second dream, where my parents gifted me a rack of elk horns, passing down this symbol of bravery, masculinity and power, entrusting me with their legacy.

FROM FEAR TO FAITH

As I let my awareness drop into the symbols in my dreams, particularly the elk as a representation of power and backbone of vitality, I couldn't help but reflect upon my generational conditioning. I started to see the bleeding elk in my dream as a symbol of my energetic depletion, while the consuming of its flesh for family dinner represented the sacrifices necessary for survival within my family lineage. It suddenly struck me that the 'no pain, no gain' attitude had been deeply ingrained in me from a young age. Memories of my grandmother surfaced in my mind, a remarkable woman who not only raised six children but also played a groundbreaking role as a physiotherapist in the 1950s. Her resilience was further echoed by her own mother, who, despite becoming a widow at a young age, managed to open her own Dairy Queen to survive. These experiences instilled in my family the belief of self-reliance.

The image of my parents passing down the elk horns portrayed the perpetuation of this generational pattern, but also served as an invitation to break free from it. From my great-grandmother to my grandma and to my mother – survival strategies passed through generations had bestowed upon me the powerful gifts of tenacity and determination. And at the same time, I realized at a deep level that working tirelessly until burnout was no longer serving my life.

In this process of going 'down and in' with the dream image, following its shadowy clues, I found the ability to integrate the lessons and gifts from my ancestors while at the same time forging my own path. The dream and the process of introspection is bringing me to a healthier relationship with productivity and success, one that doesn't sacrifice my wellbeing. While dream work is a topic that deserves its own book and is not the focus in this one, the kidneys help us to see 'down and in' to the more hidden aspects of our consciousness. They help sharpen our inner eyes to deep-seated patterns and the more abstract faculties of knowing.

Connection to ancestors and lineage

The kidneys carry both a physical and metaphysical connection to our lineage and ancestry. The *jing* essence of your kidneys is a manifestation of the collective experiences, work and survival of everyone in your lineage who came before you. Consider that even just three generations, encompassing your great-grandparents, multiply into a network of 14 unique individuals with their own hopes, fears and dreams. As you trace back even further, this network expands to include 30 people spanning four generations. Within this intricate web of genetic material and unconscious information, a wealth of ancestral connections exists, some of which you may only be partially aware of.

Different cultures demonstrate varying degrees of connection to their ancestors through storytelling and traditions. Some cultures place significant emphasis on preserving and honouring their ancestral heritage, while others, particularly those who have been colonizers, may experience a sense of disconnection from their family history and a lack of tradition. Regardless of our personal sentiments towards our ancestors or our desire to honour them, it is important to acknowledge that the kidneys carry their imprint within us as genetic memory. Our family is not something we can choose, and our physical connection to them remains unchanged. We are, in a tangible sense, a product of their existence – a reflection of the past.

Ancestors can also extend beyond our biological lineage. We can have spiritual ancestors and lineages as well. For instance, if you feel a particular affinity for Buddhism, you might carry on a certain spiritual lineage and find significance in connecting with the teachers of the past and honouring them through carrying on their teachings and practices. This spiritual dimension adds another layer to the importance of the kidneys.

Listening to a greater will

The spiritual essence of the kidneys can be compared to an acorn that carries all of the ancient information it needs to grow into a tree. Like the acorn, the kidneys hold our seed potential inherent within us, and this can be referred to as our 'entelechy'. Entelechy is not exactly equivalent to our Tao, but rather the container or framework in which our Tao takes form.

When our kidney energy is balanced on a spiritual level, we are able to listen and flow with our natural gifts, talents, abilities and idiosyncrasies instead of struggling against them. For example, you might be a naturally soft-spoken, introverted person with a great ability to listen. Feeling bad about not being more extroverted and trying to change that aspect of yourself would require a significant amount of energy. I'm not suggesting that we shouldn't challenge ourselves to grow into well-rounded individuals and work on our weaknesses, but fighting against who we are, rather than nurturing and developing our natural gifts, will deplete our life force.

While we all possess personal willpower, the universe also has its own will, known as Tian Zhi, or the 'will of heaven'. The will of heaven represents what is innate within us, our destiny and the circumstances we find ourselves in. The spiritual work of the kidneys involves aligning our personal will (our focus, attention and memory) with the will of heaven (how we were made, in combination with the larger forces at play) Through this alignment, we tap into the energy of the universe more effectively, as we are moving in the same direction as the one that the kidney essence is naturally guiding us towards. As a result, our energy is utilized more efficiently, and we often experience a stronger sense of purpose and motivation to excel in our work, engage with life and share our gifts with others.

Wisdom: 'knowing how'

Wisdom is the primary spiritual virtue associated with the kidneys, which I will define here as the skilful application of insight. It's one thing to have a profound moment of understanding during meditation, but it's another to live that understanding in your daily life. Unlike knowledge, which involves memorizing facts, wisdom is much simpler – it's about knowing what to do and how to do it, irrespective of the circumstances, in order to foster ease and balance.

The widely known 'Serenity Prayer' by Reinhold Niebuhr beautifully captures the essence of kidney wisdom: 'God, grant me the serenity to accept the things I cannot change, the courage to change the things I can, and the wisdom to know the difference.' This prayer emphasizes the kidneys' role in discerning when to surrender and rest (yin) and when to summon the courage to act (yang).

The spirit animal associated with the northern constellations of Chinese astrology embodies this wisdom held within the kidneys and water element. This unique creature is known as the 'mysterious warrior', and combines two animals into one: a blue-black tortoise intertwined with a snake.

The robust shell, long lifespan and inertia of the tortoise represents the yin principle of life preservation, steadiness and longevity of the kidney essence. Her head can retract inward when she is afraid, hiding away in her dark cave until she is ready to emerge. The tortoise's slow and deliberate movements, alongside her ability to retract deep inside herself, remind us to embrace challenges with patience and take cautious steps towards our goals. This contemplative approach encourages us to 'hide' when necessary, and to bring our attention inside to reflect before acting, enabling us to make wiser decisions and navigate life's complexities with greater clarity.

On the other hand, the snake coiling round the tortoise symbolizes the yang and masculine principle, representing the ability to extend out into the word. The snake characterizes our innate capacity to focus and narrow in on exactly what it is we want to act on. His presence signifies the importance of taking bold steps and embracing transformation in order to thrive. Additionally, the snake's winding movement and flexibility can be associated with the flow and power of our qi through meridians, representing physical vitality, health and power.

Together, the snake and tortoise represent the harmonious integration of opposing forces. They remind us of the delicate balance between rest and action, preservation and transformation, and the harmonious cooperation of yin and yang energies within ourselves.

Faith

Faith is another expression of the spirit of the kidneys and bladder when they are in balance. I am not equating faith to any blind religious belief or dogma, but rather am speaking to a deep trust that things will unfold in the right way and at the right time for your soul's development. Embodying the energy of faith means trusting that our work will yield enough resources and the belief that we are enough without needing to change who or what we are. This kind of faith arises when we listen to the inspiration from our hearts, set intentions, and diligently do the necessary work. Then, we can lean back and patiently wait for the universe to respond.

Reflecting on the symbolism of the tortoise and the snake, when the tortoise becomes pregnant, she buries her eggs in the soil, covers them up and leaves them for 70 to 120 days. She doesn't return to check on them, or sit on them, she just trusts. Her unwavering faith that they will emerge and continue her lineage encapsulates the essence of the kidneys.

One of the remarkable strengths of yin energy is the ability to stay in the dark realm of uncertainty. Faith invites us to surrender our striving when we recognize its futility, and instead trust in the natural flow of the universe for resolution.

WHERE YOU GET STUCK
WORKAHOLISM AND *JING* DEPLETION

My dream of the elk bleeding out into the shower drain alludes to a common issue many of us face: the depletion of our energy due to overwork. The 'no pain, no gain' mindset I noticed in my family line is an all-too-common phenomenon that stems from the oppression of the working class and the unsustainable expectations of modernity. It is the nature of capitalism to prioritize constant activity and negate the importance of rest and stillness. As a result, we have been conditioned to ignore the earth's natural rhythms and the rest our body needs.

It's fascinating to note that the old Roman calendar consisted of only 304 days, intentionally leaving out the remaining 61 days that fell during the winter season. There was a season to work, till the fields and know what day it was, and a season to rest. It's as if everyone was given collective permission to rest, listen and just be. While I'm not suggesting that we should do nothing for 60 days each year (although, if you have the means, I highly suggest it!), we can adopt a more mindful approach towards conserving our energy, and recognize the different seasons of the year and of our life where we may need additional time to recharge our batteries.

Remember that the kidneys hold our *jing*, which is our 'prenatal' qi, or vital essence. We only have a limited amount of *jing*, and once it is depleted, we cannot replenish it. Most of the qi we use in everyday life comes from the nourishment of the spleen and lungs. However, during long periods of stress, this energy can run dry, and we start using our *jing* reserves. *Jing* can be likened to a candle, where our spirit represents the light and the flame represents our energy. The candle is the essence or foundation of our life and once the wax is gone, so are we. Some people are born with more *jing*, like a towering pillar candle, while others have a smaller amount, like a birthday candle. These inherited qualities are known as our constitution. Those with a stronger constitution may have more energy to give and are less prone to burnout compared to those with a weaker or more fragile constitution. Nevertheless, extreme stress, pressure and overwork, regardless of your constitution, will deplete *jing* over time, leading to physical symptoms, such as premature ageing, hair loss, infertility, adrenal fatigue/chronic fatigue and back pain.

Engaging in extreme exercise, like running a marathon or participating in a triathlon, can also deplete our *jing*. According to traditional Chinese medicine, practising extreme sports that push our bodies to exhaustion on a regular basis isn't considered healthy, as it taps into our energy reserves and can potentially lead to a shorter life. However, it's important to note that this perspective doesn't consider each person's individual path or Tao. For example, if marathon running is a passion that brings you joy and uplifts your spirit, and you believe it is part of your path, it might actually benefit your energy. It's a different story altogether if you were running the marathon solely to prove yourself or to change your body shape.

Reproduction is another factor that depletes *jing*. In the case of individuals with male genitalia, each ejaculation results in *jing* loss. Retaining semen as a Taoist alchemical practice is believed to conserve life force, and practising energetic sexual yoga can allow for orgasm without losing semen. For those with female genitalia, giving birth depletes a significant amount of *jing*, as does the monthly cycle of ovulation and menstruation. Again, sexual activity and having kids is not inherently bad, as we need to sacrifice our *jing* to create new life! However, knowing that it depletes our *jing*, we can take steps to replenish the other sources of qi, such as getting adequate sleep, eating nourishing foods and being more mindful of how our energy is being expended.

Lastly, one of the fastest ways to deplete your *jing* is by striving to be someone you are not. This could show up in trying to change your core personality traits to fit into a certain relationship or career, or doing activities that 'should' be healthy, but that you really just don't have the affinity for. If you don't love yourself, you might feel like you have to take on another expression, but as a consequence the extra energy needed will drain your life force in the same way overwork will.

Fear

Our nervous system has evolved to be 'nervous' over millennia as a response to life-threatening events, such as being chased by a bear or being attacked by neighbouring village. Hormones such as adrenaline and cortisol, released in our body when we are stressed, provide us with the extra energy required to either flee or fight in such situations. However, in the 21st century, what the nervous system perceives as 'life-threatening' can take the form of an email, text message or unexpected bill; regardless of the scale of the event, our nervous systems respond similarly to how they would if we were being chased by a bear, readying us to attack or run for our lives.

It is intriguing to observe animals and their instinctual responses to recalibrate their nervous systems after experiencing a surge of stress hormones like cortisol or adrenaline. They shake their bodies to release that energy and move on. In contrast, humans tend to resort to coping mechanisms, such as watching TV, using social media or indulging in snacks. These mechanisms do not allow for the energy to resolve itself, and result in the persistent accumulation of energetic charges within our bodies, leaving our nervous systems in a state of hyperactivity. With no outlet to reset, our nervous systems are constantly overwhelmed, while the stress hormones released wreak havoc on our various critical functions, including digestion, memory and sleep.

Remembering back to Chapter 1, stress causes the Shen to flee from the nest of the heart, which causes us to lose sight of our inner truths. So, while a little fear can be helpful, constantly being overcome by fear not only leads to energetic and physical depletion, but also takes us further away from our Tao, as our mind is literally frightened out of our body.

Another consequence of consistent nervous system activation (fear) is a condition commonly referred to as 'adrenal fatigue'. Although it is not an accepted medical diagnosis, it refers to an array of symptoms, such as extreme tiredness, sleep loss, brain fog, poor memory, weight changes, hair loss and body aches, all coinciding with prolonged periods of stress. From the perspective of Chinese medicine, these symptoms are a result of kidney deficiency, because prolonged physical stress has caused the body to dip into its deep energy reserves.

On the flip side, individuals with a kidney imbalance may not experience appropriate fear, which can lead them to take unnecessary risks. It's important to note that the kidneys play a role in helping us assess risks and avoid danger, so when this energy is out of balance, it can result in reckless actions. Furthermore, those who are known as 'adrenaline junkies' and constantly seek the thrill of extreme sports, such as bungee jumping or skydiving, often exhibit signs of a kidney imbalance.

Scarcity mindset and unskilful use of resources

I have already talked about physical energetic depletion caused by stress, fear and overwork, but there are other resources that we need to conserve as well, such as time and money. Kidney imbalance can show up in the poor use of time, or in not being able to allocate time towards things that matter, as well as in squandering money or an inability to save for a rainy day. If we don't use our resources well, we can feel more stressed trying to gather them during times of need.

On the other hand, you might have enough resources, but be caught in a loop of thinking that you do not have enough. This emotion of not having enough, not being enough, not thinking your work is enough, is particularity linked to the bladder, which relates to the storage of resources. Not thinking you are enough or have enough keeps you working hard unnecessarily, and you might feel a sense of underlying urgency to do something, to save money or to hoard. It also leads you to work harder than you actually need to.

Symptoms

Take a look at the symptoms opposite, which can arise when the kidney and bladder energy are thrown off. If you notice any of these themes in your life, especially if you experience at least one symptom in each category, it might indicate that these organs need some love!'

PHYSICAL

* fatigue
* tinnitus
* hearing loss
* dark circles under the eyes
* brain fog
* hair loss
* low libido
* cold hands and feet
* insomnia
* lower back pain
* knee pain
* infertility
* frequent and/or painful urination
* osteopenia and osteoarthritis

ENERGETIC

* general forgetfulness
* inability to focus energy toward task at hand
* excessive fear and anxiety (phobias or panic attacks)
* feeling of urgency, that things need to be done NOW
* never feel like you have enough, or that you are enough
* taking unnecessary risks
* adrenaline addiction
* workaholism and pushing to the point of burnout
* poor use of resources

SPIRITUAL

* lack of will or motivation to work or complete tasks
* insecurity, lack of self-love
* low level of self-awareness
* inability to be with the unknown
* impatience
* inability to rest

SOUL WORK
FROM FEAR TO FAITH

The soul work for the kidneys invites you to re-evaluate where your energy is going. The kidneys ask you to mitigate risks and conserve resources, while not allowing fear or scarcity to rule your life. They encourage you to have faith in the unfolding of the universe, responding spontaneously and drawing upon your inherent wisdom.

Physical soul work

One of the most important things you can do for the kidneys on a physical level is to rest. Rest means physically allowing your body to stop and return the nervous system back to baseline. Slower styles of yoga that support restoration, such as yin yoga and restorative yoga, will help bring the energy more inward. Ensuring that you get enough sleep is also vital, as is recognizing that you might require more or less sleep than the 'average'. Remember, different people have different amounts of *jing*, so it is important to listen to your body when determining the amount of sleep you need. As I have mentioned in this chapter so far, our culture does not have a balanced view of what rest is. We are meant to feel guilty for not doing anything, but finding those moments of 'not doing' is essential to replenish the kidneys. Turning off the TV and electronic devices an hour before bed, as well as not engaging with your emails or activating conversations right before falling asleep, will help the nervous system unwind.

As with all organs, diet plays a big role in the health of the kidneys. Eating warm foods that are earthbound, such as root vegetables, can nourish the kidneys, as can foods that other animals store away for winter, such as nuts and seeds. Walnuts, chestnuts and black sesame are particularly nourishing for the kidneys. Eating foods that are purple and blue in colour can help too – such as blueberries, blackberries and aubergine – as well as kidney-shaped foods, like beans. It is also important to have the right amount of salt in your diet – foods like seaweed and miso can balance electrolyte levels without overdosing the body with too much sodium.

Because the bladder and kidney meridian channels move up, though and down the spine, moving your spine each day will help the qi flow through the meridians that nourish these organs and their energy. Try a simple yoga Cat/Cow pose or spinal-breathing exercise.

Lastly, the kidneys don't like to be cold! Make sure that you stay warm in winter months. Sitting or standing on cold stone or metal for long periods of time can injure the kidneys, so be sure not to expose yourself to unnecessary cold in winter, especially with the feet and spine. Applying heat to your kidneys can also help nourish them if you suspect they are out of balance in the winter months.

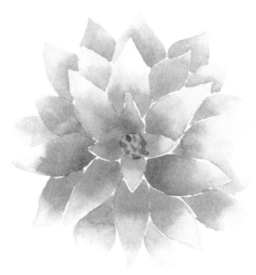

EXERCISE
SHAKING QIGONG

This practice is great for releasing fear, as well as stimulating the bones and bone marrow. If you like, you can play your favourite music to enhance the experience!

1 Stand with your feet hip-distance apart.

2 Start gently bouncing your knees up and down, allowing your whole body to shake.

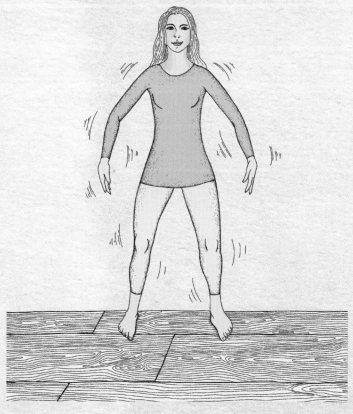

3 Once this feels comfortable, begin lifting and dropping your heels, allowing the vibration to move through your bones like a tuning fork. If your feet or legs hurt in any way, stick to bouncing with your knees.

4 Relax your internal organs while shaking and take 3–5 deep breaths, in through your nose and exhaling through your mouth.

5 Keep the bouncing motion but widen your feet to shoulder-distance apart and stop dropping the heels. Start twisting your body as you shake and allow the movement to become more free-form and improvised.

6 Gradually slow down the bouncing, close your eyes, and come to a stop. Notice how your body feels and the tingling sensations within and around it.

7 Conclude the practice with the Bringing Down the Heavens exercise (see page 58).

Energetic Soul Work

Working with the kidneys on an energetic level involves working with fear, listening to its messages and redirecting that energy into greater awareness and focus. This first involves noticing when your nervous system is in a state of activation, feeling the fear for what it is, and then applying antidotes to shift the energy.

You will notice that you are in the fear response when your heartbeat increases, your breath moves into your chest, you perhaps become shaky, dizzy, nauseous or feel disassociated from your body. Other times, 'survival mode' shows up in more subtle and chronic ways, such as not being able to sleep, deep fatigue, lower back pain, loss of appetite or loss of focus. If you suspect you have been in a fear state, or are in a fear state, take a moment to notice how it shows up in the body without it being a problem. Take a few breaths to make space around the sensation of fear, without trying to run away from it. Running from, avoiding or fighting fear, only makes it worse.

As we have learned from the energy of the lungs, there is wisdom in impulse, when it is met with awareness. Sometimes, fear is warning us of unnecessary risks, and it might be time to pull ourselves back into our shell, like the tortoise. Other times, fear might be telling you to focus your energy and act, like the snake who is ready to strike at exactly the right time.

And while fear is meant to warn you of danger, sometimes its intense exhilaration is leading you right to the growing edge of your Tao. As Marianne Williamson famously wrote, 'Our deepest fear is not that we are inadequate, but that we are powerful beyond measure.' Stepping into our own power and authenticity can be scary, especially if it is new territory. Growth usually happens at the edge of comfort. And while it is important to tread carefully at times, you would never grow if you didn't take risks and remained safe in your shell. Sometimes, it is what we are most afraid to do that is the passageway towards our most authentic and meaningful life.

Once you have felt your fear for what it is, and perhaps done the journalling activity opposite, you will need to regulate the nervous system. Just as a deer 'shakes' off to reset and walk away from her predator, you can practise the shaking qigong exercise (page 182), or heart breathing as described in Chapter 1 for a quick reset. Going for a walk and being in nature can also help discharge the overwhelming sensations of fear. Make sure you are familiar with your surroundings so that your body feels a sense of safety. Lastly, physical touch, such as a hug from a loved one or friend, or simply being with friends, can also be an invaluable way to regulate when self-applied tools are not enough.

Once the nervous system is more in a state of equilibrium, you can take the energy that has been moving through you as fear and apply it to what really matters. Remember, your time and energy are your most important resources.

'Our deepest fear is not that we are inadequate, but that we are powerful beyond measure.'

Marianne Williamson, *A Return to Love* (1992)

EXERCISE
JOURNALLING ACTIVITY

Please take out your journal or simply a pen and paper.
Set a timer for 10–15 minutes, and dedicate the time to
completing this activity and focus on nothing else. Reflect
and write about the following questions.

1 How does fear show up in your life? Is it subtle or obvious?
Is it like anxiety or panic attacks? Or is it like a low-grade
urgency? Is it a fear of not being enough or having enough?

2 What does fear feel like in your body? Does it have a shape,
colour, texture or movement? Where is it in your body?

3 What does your fear want you to know?

4 Is your fear connected somehow to a growing edge?

5 Are your resources being focused on the things that really
matter to you? Where is your energy leaking?

Spiritual Soul Work

The spiritual soul work of the kidneys is about drawing our attention inward to develop greater self-understanding and wisdom.

It is important to carve out time to allow the energy to go down and in on a regular basis, the way the tortoise pulls her body into her shell – whether that be a simple mindfulness meditation practice or a walk in solitude. Sitting by a body of water, such as an ocean, creek or river, and listening to it directly is a powerful way to nourish the kidneys and the water phase within you.

Spending time with dream images or symbols, as I did in my dream with the elk in the shower, can also open our awareness into deeper, more abstract ways of knowing, and help us understand which parts of ourselves are truly ours, and which behaviours that might have been inherited can be altered. Start a dream journal, pay attention to little coincidences and what they are telling you. Do not feel like you have to memorize the entire dream, rather keep the symbol living at the back of your mind.

Perhaps the greatest training arena for the spiritual work of the kidneys is when you are in the place of the unknown and waiting – in the place after death but before rebirth. This can be in the awkward 'in-between' phases of a project or relationship, or of something more serious, such as a cancer diagnosis or loss of a loved one. The rational mind feels safer when it feels like it knows the outcome. Rather than keeping busy to distract yourself from the discomfort of the unknown, can you allow yourself to feel tangibly into that groundlessness and what it is like? Can you surrender like a little seed and wait there patiently until something new is ready to emerge? Faith is not something that is frantic or forced, but comes in our willingness to surrender and trust in the larger unfolding of our destiny. It is an acceptance that, no matter how strong our intention is, the world often has other plans that we can never know with our rational minds. Living sanely with the world requires some level of surrender.

The development of wisdom of the kidneys is not something that happens overnight, but happens with time, as you begin to work with all the organ spirit energies and allow their messages to teach you more about the Tao and your Tao. Like water flowing down the mountain, there is more ease to how you approach your life, because you are not trying to be someone you are not. You are, in essence, embodying *wu wei*, effort without effort, moving through the world with more power, because your energy is tied to the greater force of who and what you are. You have the confidence to respond to the world and what is arising in the present moment, rather than thinking you have to control it.

EXERCISE
MEETING YOUR WISER SELF

This is a powerful meditation practice that can help bring you in touch with the part of you that already carries deep wisdom. It can be a good meditation to practise on birthdays, or if you are struggling during times that are uncertain. Seeing your life from the vantage point of the end (or the very beginning) can help highlight what really matters to you and where your energy is best spent.

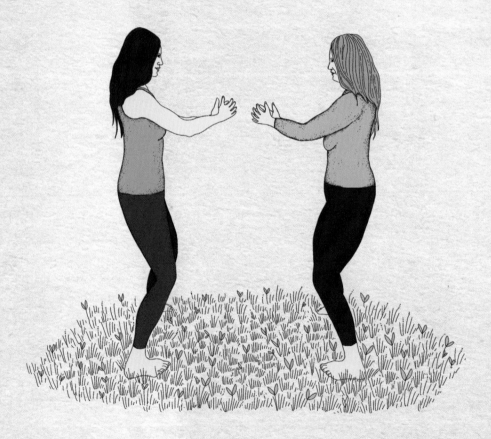

1 Begin by finding a comfortable position, whether seated or lying down. Take a few deep breaths and let your entire body relax.

2 Once you feel safe enough to do so, visualize a horizon line that represents the balance of yin and yang energies, where the heavens and earth meet. Take a few moments to surrender into that energy.

3 Next, imagine a version of yourself that is older and wiser. You might see yourself at the very end of your life. Maybe you are 84, or 104. Take a moment to truly observe this wise being and notice how you feel in their presence. Look deep into their eyes.

4 If this doesn't feel right to you, you could also imagine yourself at the very beginning of your life, as an infant, as these beings are wise too! It is said we are closest to our most authentic self at birth and before death.

5 Once you have a clear image or 'felt sense' of this being, ask what it wants you to know. You may seek insights into the most important aspects of your life, where your energy should be focused, or what truly matters to you. Remember that this wise being may communicate with you through images, symbols or body sensations, rather than spoken language.

6 Allow yourself some time to connect deeply with this wise being, and, once you feel ready, take a moment to journal any messages or symbols that felt significant.

CONCLUSION

We are not separate from this Earth;
we are a part of it, whether we fully
feel it in our bodies yet or not.
It's a contract you see, people and the land.

You care for it, and it cares for you.

Sharon Blackie, *If Women Rose Rooted*

look up at the brightening night sky, its blue hues signalling the return of daylight. Early morning stars greet my waking eyes and I gaze back intimately, as I would a lover. It's been four days of fasting solo in the Arizona desert, accompanied by the presence of javelinas and crows. I've grown acquainted with the red mountains, the towering saguaros that stand guard over my camp, and the moon that illumes my dreams and night vision. Despite the ice coating my sleeping bag, I am warm within it, and relax my organs towards my spine. I let my limbs extend out and merge into the desert floor. As I feel my tailbone ground into the earth, I am reminded that, while I am not actually a part of the land, I am undoubtedly an animal, wild, like the javelina. 'It is difficult to be a creature,' I muse.

In these few days, I have witnessed creatures around me engage in their relentless battles for food and staunch guardianship over precious water sources. Even the plants have adapted defence mechanisms, with sharp spikes protecting their flesh from thirsty birds. And yet, there is wisdom in their impulse – to know when a storm is coming and how to survive by drawing water from sand and stones, and in doing so maintain balance within the ecosystem, each species playing a role in desert life unfolding. I think of humans, like cacti erecting their spikes of protection, and competing for resources in our concrete jungles. Somewhere along the line, it seems we have forgotten about balance.

As the stars fade above me, I am reminded of the other part of our nature – one that has foresight and vision, that can create and love, that is self-aware and wonders about the mysteries of life and death. Like the stars, we have a wider perspective and can see what lies beyond the desert terrain.

Lying in the dirt I feel my animal self and my starlight self in conversation. My back embraced by the yin, my front open to yang, and my soul dancing somewhere in between. If I neglect the light, I am the boar running wild. If I neglect my animal body, I live in the sky as light disengaged from the vitality that sustains life. What would it be like for that light to guide the wisdom of this body? What gifts would be remembered so I can step in rhythm with the earth and what she needs?

The sun crests over the mountain, and its beam touches my face. I close my eyes and absorb it. While I do not yet know the details of my way, I feel an impulse to move confidently into the next step of the journey.

Next steps

I hope this book has sparked a conversation between your starlight self and your animal self, and has provided insights into different areas of your body, energy and mind that could benefit from your attention and care. Now that you have completed this journey through your organs, I encourage you to continue exploring them. Following your Tao is a lifelong practice that is never truly 'complete', but rather an ongoing process of growth and discovery. Your body's wisdom is instinctive and spontaneous, always responding to the present moment. Sometimes, when we learn something new and feel excited about it, we tend to plan ahead. However, I encourage you to stay present and focus on the next simple step. It's absolutely okay if you don't have all the answers right now. In fact, if you have more questions than you did before reading this book, that is great news! Curiosity is the fuel for continued learning and self-discovery.

Following your Tao is not about escaping the pain that is naturally bound up with human life, but rather is about creatively engaging with it. Trying to escape the realities of pain and loss is akin to attempting to be a star in the sky. Instead, this book provides a different way to relate to your animal body and its suffering. I hope it will continue to prompt you to explore different perspectives on your pain, and rather than looking at your body as a machine that has failed you, you can stay open to what it might be trying to say.

Most importantly, this book is not meant to gather dust on your shelf; it's intended as a resource you can return to repeatedly. Please mark it up, dog ear it, flag it – keep it as a companion. For example, during a season of loss in your life, turning to the lung chapter might guide you deeper into its wisdom. If you're feeling anger, jealousy or guilt, consulting the liver chapter would be helpful. My hope is that this book helps you to speak the language of the five spirits and to proactively balance your energy.

In addition to the exercises outlined in this book, I highly encourage practising sitting somewhere familiar in nature without a specific agenda or predetermined destination. Simply sit and engage in a conversation with the surrounding environment. The opening narratives in each chapter serve as examples of how this way of just being and observing nature can provide direct insights. While I don't expect you to spend four days in the desert fasting, I do encourage experiencing nature as directly as possible, without the distraction of headphones, cellphones or other electronic devices. Even if you live in a city, you can still connect to nature through elements like the sun, rain, bees and birds. Alternatively, you can use your imagination to connect with nature if that feels safer or more accessible to you.

When engaging in this practice of sitting in nature, remember that all relationships are reciprocal. If you feel called to, you can also give back to that place in some way. It could be offering something to the land, such as a flower, sage or tobacco. It could also be as simple as picking up a piece of garbage. Alternatively, you can express your gratitude through a song, a prayer or something that gives back in your own unique way.

Relearning enoughness

What I have noticed about teaching programmes in the five organ energies is that they often have a deeper effect on people's lives than they initially expect. What starts as a curiosity about the organs, turns into discovery of one's own authentic expression. The white tiger's defence mechanisms are relaxed, and one's Tao starts to rush forward into conscious awareness. For some, the impact of this manifests in a renewed focus on their art, allowing their creativity to flourish. Others may find the courage to pursue their passion by leaving their current jobs and embarking on a new path. There are also those who experience a more internal transformation, shifting the way they relate to themselves or their family. Some people learn to set boundaries, and others have more of a quiet appreciation for everyday moments. Remember that your Tao is not necessarily what you do, and the changes you make do not have to be grandiose, nor do they have to do with a vocation or making money. Growing into your authentic expression is a way of being that gives back – like the water that flows down the mountain.

Be on the lookout for self-doubt and imposter syndrome – a common phenomenon in our modern world that has taught us that our self-worth relates to money and external validation. Capitalism has taught us that our value needs to be accredited by an institution, university or course. Please let me tell you this: no course, university, certification, number of social media followers or amount of money will 'approve' the gifts that lie within you. Imposter syndrome is an expression of mistrusting your own gifts, and on a wider universal level, mistrusting the gifts of the earth.

Even if you practise none of the exercises outlined in this book, know that simply directing your awareness to your breath brings harmony to your Shen and Po, balancing your upper spirits with the lower. When you set a boundary with a co-worker, you are protecting the energy of your heart. When you are compassionate to yourself, you are exercising the virtue of your liver, and while completing tasks on your to-do list you nurture your spleen. When you rest, you can think of your kidneys thanking you as you drift off into the world of dreams. Let what you have read inspire a deep appreciation for the intelligences inside you, and how they have supported your life journey so far. Understanding this alone holds its own value, and adopting this way of listening can guide you back to your Tao.

A Parting Prayer

May your heart guide you towards the truth of who you are. May joy expand you into a wider circle of connection, where your light can be seen and celebrated.

May your liver move you in the direction of your dreams, giving you the tenacity to stand up for the benefit of all. May compassion hold you in your imperfection, patiently supporting you in your growth.

May your spleen centre your resolve in each steady step of the journey, grounding your intentions with constancy into your thoughts, words and actions. May you remember earth as your original mother and allow yourself to fully receive her nourishment.

May your lungs hold on to what is precious, and help you release when the time is right. May grief act as a teacher for deeper love and understanding of what it means to be mortal.

May your kidneys instil faith in the fertile darkness, helping you navigate the unknown. May fear help safeguard your resources and challenge you to emerge into your most authentic expression.

INDEX

BIBLIOGRAPHY

Ardiel, E.L. and Rankin, C.H. 'The Importance of Touch in Development', Paediatrics and Child Health, vol. 15(3), pp. 153–6. Oxford University Press, 2010.

Cadegiani, F.A. and Kater, C.E. 'Adrenal Fatigue Does Not Exist: A Systematic Review', BMC Endocrine Disorders, vol. 16(1). National Library of Medicine, 2016.

Chia, Mantak, and Winn, Michael. *Taoist Secrets of Love: Cultivating Male Sexual Energy.* Aurora Press, 1984.

Cohen, Kenneth. 'Medical Qigong: Fact or Fiction?' *Journal of Scientific Exploration*, vol. 28, No. 1, pp. 176–187, 2014.

Cohen, Kenneth. *The Way of Qigong: the Art and Science of Chinese Energy Healing.* Ballantine Books, 1999.

Dechar, Lorie Eve and Fox, Benjamin. *The Alchemy of Inner Work: A Guide for Turning Illness and Suffering into True Health and Well-Being.* Red Wheel/Weiser, 2021.

Dechar, Lorie Eve. *Five Spirits: Alchemical Acupuncture for Psychological and Spiritual Healing.* Lantern Books, 2005.

Dechar, Lorie Eve. Kigo: *Exploring the Spiritual Essence of Acupuncture Points Through the Changing Seasons.* Singing Dragon, 2020.

Dunbar, R. I. (2010). 'The Social Role of Touch in Humans and Primates: Behavioural Function and Neurobiological Mechanisms.' *Neuroscience & Biobehavioral Reviews*, 34(2), 260-268.

Epstein, Mark. *The Trauma of Everyday Life.* Penguin Books, 2014.

Field, T. 'Touch for Socioemotional and Physical Well-being: A Review', *Developmental Review*, vol. 30(4), pp. 367–83. Elsevier, 2010.

Fischer, Norman. *The World Could Be Otherwise: Imagination and the Bodhisattva Path.* Shambhala, 2019.

Fronsdal, Gil. *The Issue at Hand: Essays on Buddhist Mindfulness Practice.* Insight Meditation Center, 2008.

Gliga, T., Farroni, T., & Cascio, C. J. (2019). 'Social Touch: A New Vista For Developmental Cognitive Neuroscience?. *Developmental Cognitive Neuroscience*, 35, 1-4.

Haim-Litevsky, D., Komemi, R. and Lipskaya-Velikovsky, L. 'Sense of Belonging, Meaningful Daily Life Participation and Well-being: Integrated Investigation', *International Journal of Environmental Research and Public Health*, vol. 20(5), p. 4121. National Library of Medicine, 2023.

Hanh, Thich Nhat. *The Miracle of Mindfulness*. Beacon Press, 1996.

Hanh, Thich Nhat. *Silence: The Power of Quiet in a World Full of Noise*. Rider, 2015.

Hanson, Rick. *Hardwiring Happiness*. Rider, 2014.

Hanson, Rick and Mendius, Richard. *Buddha's Brain: The Practical Neuroscience of Happiness, Love and Wisdom*. New Harbinger, 2009.

Harper, Douglas. Online Etymology Dictionary: www.etymonline.com

HeartMath Institute Research Library: www.heartmath.org/research/research-library

Johnson, Jerry Alan. *The Secret Teachings of Chinese Energetic Medicine, vols. 1–5*. The International Institute of Medical Qigong Publishing House, 2014.

Jung, Carl. *Man and His Symbols*. Bantam, 2023.

Jung, Carl and Wilhelm, Richard. *The Secret of the Golden Flower*. Martino, 2014.

Kirkwood, John. *The Way of the Five Seasons: Living with Five Elements for Physical, Emotional and Spiritual Harmony*. Singing Dragon, 2016.

Kirkwood, John. *The Way of the Five Elements: 52 Weeks of Powerful Acupoints for Physical, Emotional and Spiritual Health*. Singing Dragon, 2008.

Kittisaro and Thanissara. *Listening to the Heart: A Contemplative Journey to Engaged Buddhism*. North Atlantic Books, 2014.

Kornfield, Jack. *The Wise Heart: A Guide to the Universal Teachings of Buddhist Psychology*. Bantam, 2009.

Kuo-Deemer, Mimi. *Qigong and the Tai Chi Axis: Nourishing Practices for Body, Mind and Spirit*. Ixia Press, 2019.

Larre, Claude and Rochat de la Vallee, Elisabeth. *The Secret Treatise of the Spiritual Orchid: Nei Jing Su Wen Chapter 8*. Monkey Press, 2014.

Levine, Glenn N., et al. 'Psychological Health, Well-Being and the Mind-Heart-Body Connection: A Scientific Statement from the American Heart Association', *Circulation*, vol. 143(10). AHA Journals, 2021.

Lo, Vi and Yidan, W. 'Chasing the Vermilion Bird: Late Medieval Alchemical Transformations in the Treasure Book of Ilkhan on Chinese Science and Techniques', *Imagining Chinese Medicine*, vol. 18, pp. 291–304. Brill, 2018.

Macarenco, M, et al. 'Childhood Trauma, Dissociation, Alexithymia and Anger in People with Autoimmune Diseases: A Mediation Model', *Child Abuse and Neglect*, vol. 122, p.105322. National Library of Medicine, 2021.

Machado de Oliveira, Vanessa. *Hospicing Modernity: Parting with Harmful Ways of Living*. North Atlantic Books, 2021.

McCraty R, et al. 'Phasic Induction of Bioelectromagnetic Heart-Brain Coupling through Emotional Stimuli,' *Journal of Xi'an Shiyou University, Natural Science Edition*, vol. 19(4). Research Library Publication, 2023.

'Matthew McConaughey Motivational Speech Transcript', 7 January 2016: www.rev.com.

Mead, Daniel F. 'If You Would Grow', as posted by Renée Bochman on Compassion Camp: https://compassioncamp.com

Meade, Michael. *Fate and Destiny: The Two Agreements of the Soul*. Greenfire Press, 2012.

Meade, Michael. *The Genius Myth*. Seattle: Greenfire Press, 2016.

Meade, Michael. 'The Path We Are Trying to Find: Ego Re-education and the Original Purpose of Fear', on the podcast *Love & Liberation with Olivia Clementine*, 18 November 2021.

Mojay, Gabriel. *Aromatherapy for Healing the Spirit: Psychological and Energetic Aspects of Essential Oils*. Hodder Headline, 1996.

Oliver, Mary. *American Primitive: Poems*. Back Bay Books, 1984.

Narvaez, D., Wang, L., Cheng, A., Gleason, T. R., Woodbury, R., Kurth, A., & Lefever, J. B. (2019). 'The Importance of Early Life Rouch for Psychosocial and Moral Development'. *Psicologia: Reflexão e Crítica*, 32, 16.

Plotkin, Bill. *Soulcraft: Crossing into the Mysteries of Nature and Psyche*. New World Library, 2003.

Plotkin, Bill. *Wild Mind: A Field Guide to the Human Psyche*. New World Library, 2013.

Powers, Sarah. *Insight Yoga: An Innovative Synthesis of Traditional Yoga, Meditation, and Eastern Approaches to Healing and Well-Being*. Shambhala Publications, 2009.

Powers, Sarah. *Lit from Within: Yoga, Teachings, and Practices to Illuminate Our Inner Lives*. Shambhala Publications, 2021.

Qicheng, Z., Jing, W. and Dear, D. 'Embodying Animal Spirits in the Vital Organs: Daoist Alchemy in Chinese Medicine', *Imagining Chinese Medicine*, pp. 389–96. Brill, 2018.

Robinson, Bryan E. 'The 90-Second Rule That Builds Self-Control', *Psychology Today*, 26 April 2020.

Sakakibara, M. 'Evaluation of Heart Rate Variability and Application of Heart Rate Variability Biofeedback: Toward Further Research on Slow-Paced Abdominal Breathing in Zen Meditation', *Applied Psychophysiology and Biofeedback*, vol. 47(4) pp. 345–56. National Library of Medicine, 2022.

Salihoğlu, S, Doğan, S. C., and Kavakçı, Ö. 'Effects of Childhood Psychological Trauma on Rheumatic Diseases', *European Journal of Rheumatology*, vol. 6(3), pp. 126–9. National Library of Medicine, 2019.

Schwartz, Richard C. *No Bad Parts: Healing Trauma and Restoring Wholeness with the Internal Family Systems Model*. Sounds True, 2021.

Shadick, N. A., et al. 'A Randomized Controlled Trial of an Internal Family Systems-Based Psychotherapeutic Intervention on Outcomes in Rheumatoid Arthritis: A Proof-of-Concept Study', *The Journal of Rheumatology*, vol. 40(11). National Library of Medicine, 2013.

Sharpe, L. 'Psychosocial Management of Chronic Pain in Patients with Rheumatoid Arthritis: Challenges and Solutions'. *Journal of Pain Research*, 137-146, 2016.

Smith, Huston and Novak, Philip. *Buddhism: A Concise Introduction*. HarperCollins, 2005.

Tara Brach's Dharma Talks: https://dharmaseed.org

Taylor, Jill Bolte. *My Stroke of Insight*. Penguin, 2008.

Tzu, Lao and Mitchell, Stephen. *Tao Te Ching: A New English Version*. Harper & Row, 1989.

Watkins, E.R., and Roberts, H. 'Reflecting on Rumination: Consequences, Causes, Mechanisms and Treatment of Rumination', *Behaviour Research and Therapy*, vol. 127(1). National Library of Medicine, 2020.

Williamson, Marianne. *A Return to Love*. Thorsons, 1996.

RESOURCES & FURTHER READING

Five Elements, Chinese Medicine & Taoism

Abbs, Ashey. *5 Element Alchemy: Use Your 5 Element Type to Embrace Your Gifts and Create a Life You Love.* Embodied Elements Press, 2021.

Choi, Lily and Koutroumanis, Bess. *Heal Yourself with Traditional Chinese Medicine: Find Relief from Chronic Pain, Stress, Hormonal Issues and More with Natural Practices and Ancient Knowledge.* Page Street Publishing, 2023.

Dechar, Lorie Eve. *The Five Spirits: Alchemical Acupuncture for Psychological and Spiritual Healing.* Lantern Books, 2006.

Dechar, Lorie Eve and Fox, Benjamin. *The Alchemy of Inner Work: A Guide for Turning Illness and Suffering into True Health and Well-Being.* Red Wheel/Weiser, 2021.

Hoff, Benjamin. *The Tao of Pooh.* Farshore, 2018.

Kirkwood, John. *The Way of the Five Seasons: Living with the Five Elements for Physical, Emotional and Spiritual Harmony.* Singing Dragon, 2016.

Mitchel, Stephen. *The Tao Te Ching.* Harper Collins, 1992.

Qigong

Cohen, Kenneth. *The Way of Qigong: the Art and Science of Chinese Energy Healing.* Ballantine Books, 1999.

Jwing Ming, Dr Yang. *The Root of Chinese Qigong: Secrets for Health, Longevity and Enlightenment.* YMA, 1997.

Kuo-Deemer, Mimi. *Qigong and the Tai Chi Axis: Nourishing Practices for Body, Mind and Spirit.* Orion Spring, 2018.

Nosco, Stephanie: Online courses to learn qigong, visit www.stephanienosco.com

Mindfulness

Feldman, Christina. *Boundless Heart: The Buddha's Path of Kindness, Compassion, Joy and Equanimity.* Shambhala, 2017.

Fronstal, Gil. *The Issue at Hand.* Download and read for free here: www.insightmeditationcenter.org/books-articles/the-issue-at-hand/

Gunaratana, Bhante Bhante. *Mindfulness in Plain English: 20th Anniversary Edition.* Wisdom Publications, 2011.

Hanh, Thich Nhat. *The Miracle of Mindfulness.* Rider, 2008.

Kittisaro and Thanissara. *Listening to the Heart: A Contemplative Journey to Engaged Buddhism.* North Atlantic Books, 2014.

Kornfield, Jack. *The Wise Heart: A Guide to the Universal Teachings of Buddhist Psychology.* Rider, 2008.

Powers, Sarah. *Insight Yoga: An Innovative Synthesis of Traditional Yoga, Meditation, and Eastern Approaches to Healing and Well-Being.* Shambhala Publications, 2009.

Nutrition & Herbs

Ashton, Kimberly: Qi Food Therapy online webinars, cookbooks and courses, visit https://www.qifoodtherapy.com, or follow @qifoodtherapy

Goldsmith, Ellen and Klein, Maya. *Nutritional Healing with Chinese Medicine.* Robert Rose, 2017.

Superfeast Podcast and Chinese Herbs: https://superfeast.com

Dream Work

Book of Symbols, The. Taschen, 2022.

Johnson, Robert. *Inner Work: Using Dreams and Active Imagination for Personal Growth.* Harper San Francisco, 1991.

Johnson, Robert. *Owning Your Own Shadow: Understanding the Dark Side of the Psyche.* Bravo, 1994.

Plotkin, Bill. *Soulcraft: Crossing into the Mysteries of Nature and Psyche.* New World Library, 2003.

Sowton, Christopher. *Dreamworking: How to Listen to the Inner Guidance of Your Dreams.* Llewellyn, 2017.

This Jungian Life, Podcast and Dream School: https://thisjungianlife.com

Toko-pa Turner Dream School, visit https://toko-pa.com/dreamschool/

Essential Oils and Acupressure

Dechar, Lorie Eve. *Kigo: Exploring the Spiritual Essence of Acupuncture Points Through the Changing Seasons.* Singing Dragon, 2020.

Kirkwood, John. *The Way of the Five Elements: 52 Weeks of Powerful Acupoints for Physical, Emotional and Spiritual Health.* Singing Dragon, 2018.

Mojay, Gabriel. *Aromatherapy for Healing the Spirit: Restoring Emotional and Mental Balance with Essential Oils.* Healing Arts Press, 2000.

ABOUT THE AUTHOR

Stephanie Nosco is a qigong teacher, psychotherapist, educator, writer and creative based on Vancouver Island, Canada. For over 15 years, Stephanie has dedicated herself to guiding individuals into their inner world through movement and meditation practices. She has two arts degrees in Religious Studies and Education, complemented by a master's in Counselling Psychology. Stephanie's teachings are a unique blend of meditation, yin yoga and qigong, which she enjoys sharing on the retreats and online programs she offers to a worldwide audience.

In her psychotherapy practice, Stephanie employs an eclectic approach, integrating depth psychology, Buddhist psychology and intuitive energetics. As a lifelong learner, she is deeply committed to her own path of self-discovery and earnestly embodies the practices she teaches.

Explore more about Stephanie's online courses and retreats at her website, www.stephanienosco.com. For daily doses of inspiration, follow her Instagram page, @stephanienosco.

ACKNOWLEDGEMENTS

This book owes its existence to the majestic Rocky Mountains, ancient old-growth forests and expansive prairie skies. I want to express my heartfelt appreciation for my home province of Alberta, Canada, which lies on the traditional lands of the Siksika, Kainai and Piikani First Nations, the Tsuut'ina Nation and Métis Region 3. And thank you to the land I currently reside on, in beautiful British Columbia, which is the traditional and unceded territory of the Coast Salish people, particularly the Snuneymuxw, Qualicum and Snaw-Naw-As First Nations.

I would also like to extend my deepest gratitude to my teachers, Sarah and Ty Powers, who served as my main guides in the exploration of the Buddha Dharma and energetic practices. A special thank you goes to Carly Forest, who offered invaluable mentorship during challenging times on retreat and introduced me to medical qigong. Additionally, I express my sincerest appreciation to Wendy Lang, my instructor in medical qigong and shamanic Chinese medicine. Thank you to Lorie Dechar and Benjamin Fox, who not only taught me the language of the Five Spirits but also embodied a profound commitment to upholding a vibrant community of healers. Gratitude is also owed to Thanissara and Kitisaro, my Buddhist teachers, and all the teachers at Spirit Rock who guided and supported me during the early stages of rediscovering myself. I offer a heartfelt shout-out to Ashley Abbs, whose unwavering mentorship and belief in my emerging voice made this book possible.

I would also like to express my sincerest appreciation to my assistant, Colleen, who aided me in drafting the initial book proposal and supported my work throughout the writing process. Thank you, Jon, for nurturing my growth as a pathfinder, and Christine, for providing discerning listening and ongoing support from the beginning. I extend my thanks to all my supportive friends (particularly Emmaly, Catherine and Adam), students and followers who cheered me along the way.

Lastly, my deepest gratitude goes to my parents, Marie and Steve Babcock, and to my partner, Ben, and our feline companion, Kirby, for their unwavering support while I immersed myself in the process of writing this book. Your love and understanding made all the difference.

Stephanie

All original images by Bethan Christopher, www.bethanchristopher.com. Other images courtesy of Shutterstock:/ 9comeback 9 / Anna Holyph 151 / ArtMari 4 / Artnizu 73, 88 / Creative_Captain 116 / Domira 149 / Julia August 16 / kitouL 101 / Kjpargeter 6–7, 26–6 / ledokolua 131 / Marina Demidova 12, 48, 96, 115, 182 / marukopum 20–21 / Rudchenko Liliia 29, 45, 77, 81, 123, 141, 157, 165, 186 / Tasefa Design 71 / Valedi 163 / VerisStudio 8, 14, 57, 111, 146, 180, 189, 192, 196, 207.